The Undreaded Job

Recent Titles in
International Contributions in Psychology

The Undreaded Job

Learning to Thrive in a Less-than-Perfect Workplace

RICHARD BRISLIN

International Contributions in Psychology
Paul Pedersen, Series Editor

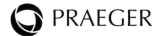

PRAEGER

AN IMPRINT OF ABC-CLIO, LLC
Santa Barbara, California • Denver, Colorado • Oxford, England

Library of Congress Cataloging-in-Publication Data
Brislin, Richard.
  The undreaded job : learning to thrive in a less-than-perfect workplace / Richard Brislin.
    p. cm. — (International contributions in psychology)
  Includes bibliographical references and index.
  ISBN 978-0-313-38591-9 (hard copy : alk. paper)—ISBN 978-0-313-38592-6 (ebook)
1. Quality of work life. 2. Work—Psychological aspects. 3. Work environment.
4. Employees—Attitudes. 5. Organizational behavior. 6. Interpersonal relations. I. Title.
  HD6955.B735 2010
  650.1—dc22   2010003458

ISBN: 978-0-313-38591-9
EISBN: 978-0-313-38592-6

14 13 12 11 10   1 2 3 4 5

This book is also available on the World Wide Web as an eBook.
Visit www.abc-clio.com for details.

Praeger
An Imprint of ABC-CLIO, LLC

ABC-CLIO, LLC
130 Cremona Drive, P.O. Box 1911
Santa Barbara, California 93116-1911

This book is printed on acid-free paper ∞

Manufactured in the United States of America

Copyright Acknowledgments

Much of the information within this book was first published in articles written for the *Honolulu Star-Bulletin*.

Contents

Series Foreword

I grew up on an Iowa farm where the work was endless. My father always reminded me that "work" was God's greatest blessing, but I never understood what he meant until I was an adult and came to appreciate how precious work can be. Brislin's book does a good job of capturing the precious value of work in giving our life meaning, both in measuring our self-satisfaction and our satisfactoriness in the eyes of others. Now that I am retired, strangers ask me what I do and when I reply that I am retired, the next question is often, "What did you do when you had a job?" Brislin's book describes the ways our work role gives our life meaning.

The genius of each chapter is grounding each practical application in a theoretical understanding of psychological research. For example, is good management a necessary but not sufficient condition for good leadership? In our organizational skills, what are the consequences of answering questions that have not been asked? Our career is, in some ways, like buying a house. "I can't tell you what I want, but I will recognize it when I see it." In our workplace roles we need to avoid "scratching where it doesn't itch." What you hear might be quite different from what I say. A little knowledge about the workplace might be dangerous in providing enough knowledge to make a fluent fool of yourself. The key to power in the workplace is to make the job easier for your employers. In our analysis of workplace attitudes, no matter how different another group might seem there are always similarities, and no matter how similar they might seem there are always differences. This book will help you identify the diversity in each context, which is just as necessary to a healthy organization as biological diversity is necessary for promoting a healthy gene pool for the perpetuation of a species.

The Brislin book fits well with the International Contributions in Psychology series, describing how psychological services are of practical value across boundaries of countries and cultures. The many books in this series define the cutting edge of psychology as applied to social issues. Each book has focused on a specific social issue of importance, providing building blocks to those who deliver psychological services to an informed society. It is with great pride that we welcome this most recent contribution to the series.

Paul Pedersen
Professor Emeritus, Syracuse University
Series Editor

1

Introduction: Finding Happiness in the Workplace

Finding satisfaction, self-efficacy, and a sense of self-fulfillment in the workplace is one of the most important factors contributing to a sense of happiness and contentment with life (Diener & Seligman, 2004). Put alternatively, dissatisfaction with work contributed to discontent, and this often spills over into other aspects of people's lives such as relations with family members and friends (Blustein, 2006). The purpose of this book is to draw from research in psychology, management, and related fields to give people information that should help them find more satisfaction with their work lives.

Consider the benefits that success in the workplace can bring. The workplace is a place where people have positive social interactions with others. It is a place where people find a sense of identity that contributes to the self-view that they are worthwhile people. The workplace is one of the venues where people achieve social status that affects how they are treated in other arenas of life such as their communities and churches. It is a place where some people meet their life partners. The workplace provides an income that allows people to support themselves and other family members. It can provide other tangible benefits such as medical insurance and a retirement plan (Noe, Hollenbeck, Gerhart, & Wright, 2008). Occasionally, perhaps less often than 50 years ago, it can provide a sense of security that people will always have a job, an income, and the status accompanying holding down a job. The workplace can provide other benefits such as travel, opportunities for advanced training, and exposure to the knowledge and skills of cooperative colleagues.

With the possible exception of sleeping, most people will spend more time working than they will spend on any other activity. People can get up in the morning and be pleased about going to work because of the interesting challenges they will face and the cooperative colleagues with whom they will interact. If people travel during a three-week vacation, they can look forward to coming back to work on the eighteenth or nineteenth day of their trips. They can view their work as central to their identity and can be proud of their answers when people ask, "What do you do?"

I have great sympathy for people who do not like their work. I meet such people when I interact in various community volunteer groups. Some people I know despise their work. They get up in the morning and dread getting into their cars and commuting to their workplaces. They can generate no enthusiasm for the tasks that face them on a given day. They talk about changing jobs but often cannot because they do not have the qualifications called for in other job announcements. Further, they often have family commitments that affect their career mobility (Lazarova & Lowe, 2008). They cannot afford to take time off from their jobs to further their education and to obtain the skills necessary for more attractive work.

A key to lifetime happiness, then, is finding work that one enjoys. Parents and educators often guide adolescents and young adults into intelligent choices concerning work. Parents advise their children to volunteer for different types of community activities to see what aspects of work they enjoy. Educators advise students to undertake internships in companies to determine if certain types of jobs are suitable given their personalities, abilities, and values.

Throughout this book, I will try to contribute to people's enjoyment of their work by discussing various issues that lead to a greater understanding of leadership, power, motivation, group dynamics, social skills, and other topics central to an understanding of human behavior in organizations. Many times, people cannot change any of these aspects of their organizations. Certain superiors have an irritating leadership style, certain groups seem to exclude newcomers, and some coworkers seem to become intoxicated whenever they are given a little power. However, workplace tensions will often decrease if people increase their understanding of why these concepts are important, how different individuals apply them with greater and less amounts of success, and what long-term outcomes are likely to be (Bandura, 2001). Put another way, people can increase their workplace satisfaction if they understand basic concepts surrounding such workplace issues as leadership, groups, and power (Brislin, 1991). They can apply their knowledge of workplace concepts to their organizations and have the satisfaction of understanding what is happening, even if they cannot change it immediately. I hope to give advice that will help people encourage changes when these are possible, accept the quirks of others when change is not an option, and increase their chances of increasing their job sophistication so that they will occasionally win office battles with those who are causing workplace unhappiness.

2

Leadership

INTRODUCTION

If new hires in an organization are fortunate, they will receive good mentoring advice from their wiser elders who have been members of the workforce for 10 or more years. One specific piece of wisdom is, "It is your job to get along with your boss, not your boss's job to get along with you. Bosses are just too busy to have to spend time figuring out how to get along with each of their subordinates."

I hope young hires take this advice seriously. Bosses have many responsibilities, and if subordinates can help with those responsibilities and at the same time demonstrate a cooperative and positive attitude, their careers are likely to advance. Consider just a few of the responsibilities that bosses have to undertake. They must set the directions of their organizations or the directions of the divisions which they head. Bosses must communicate what they expect of their subordinates so that everyone's efforts can contribute to organizational goals. They must model appropriate workplace activities and must "walk the talk," not just tell people what to do but demonstrate actual desirable workplace behaviors. Bosses must identify and nurture their most talented employees to ensure effective leaders in the future. They must be a positive representative of their organization in their communities and bring positive attention to their workplace through various volunteer activities (Kinicki & Williams, 2008). There are other activities expected of bosses that will be covered in various chapters of this book.

Employees will be aided in their efforts to get along with their bosses, and to contribute to accomplishing the company goals set by their bosses, if they are aware of the expectations the bosses are expected to fulfill. These expectations can be set by company presidents, boards of directors, customers, and (in the case of governmental positions) the electorate. A good start to understanding the role of boss is to examine various terms that summarize their responsibilities. Two terms frequently used, and sometimes used interchangeably, are *manager* and *leader*.

Management and Leadership Are Necessary in the Workplace

Having graduated with a degree in engineering, Mike Yamasato went to work for a construction firm in Honolulu five years ago. Until recently, he had been under the supervision of different engineers who were 10 to 15 years older. Last week, he received a promotion to a position where he would supervise a staff of 12 people. Some of his old bosses congratulated him and added, "Welcome to the ranks of management." At his first meeting with other supervisors, most of the discussion dealt with different leadership issues. Not having taken business courses in college, Mike was unclear about the distinctions between management and leadership.

Mike's confusion is understandable since *management* and *leadership* are words that are often used interchangeably. When careful distinctions are made, management is the broader term. Managers plan for the future and take steps to ensure that the necessary information is available for good decision making. They organize the people over whom they have supervisory responsibilities and make certain that procedures are in place for hiring, staff development, promotions, and communications with potential customers. They oversee control procedures to ensure that projects are completed on schedule and that customers are being given the highest-quality work possible. Managers also lead people, taking people in directions that will benefit them and the company for which they work.

Leadership is often the most discussed aspect of management (Kinicki & Williams, 2008; Yukl, 2010). Leadership issues arise most often in times of rapid change, increased competition, and major changes in a community's economic outlook. Leaders take followers in new directions toward goals that are set through participatory decision making. Often, a leader's subordinates would not work toward these goals unless the leader communicated a clear vision of a desirable future that will bring benefits to all workers in a company. Leaders must have the highly desirable skills of communicating clearly with followers and instilling confidence that the goals are achievable if all work together. Leaders must earn the trust of followers when they say,

"Hitch your wagon to the star that I visualize and we will all reap benefits."

Both good management and good leadership are necessary. Management tasks may not seem as glamorous but they are essential to the smooth functioning of a company. Examples include meeting payrolls, pairing new hires with experienced workers who are willing to be mentors, and responding to office memos in a timely fashion. At times, charismatic leaders with an inspired vision are not successful because of inattention to the everyday tasks of managers. In such cases, leaders should have the self-insight to recognize their weaknesses and should take appropriate steps. For example, they might hire strong administrative assistants who can carry out assigned managerial tasks that the leaders themselves might mishandle.

TASK AND SOCIAL ASPECTS OF LEADERSHIP

The research literature on leadership in private-sector organizations, education, and politics is extensive (Aycan, 2008; Judge, Ilies, & Colbert, 2004; Van Vugt, Hogan, & Kaiser, 2008; Yukl, 2010), and provides a wealth of helpful advice. Researchers who have devoted years of their careers to the study of leadership often develop theories that allow the work of leaders to be described and to assess their effectiveness. Every theory of leadership contains the requirement that managers and executives balance the task and the social aspects of leadership. Task aspects include hiring good employees, overseeing the production of high-quality products and services, meeting consumer demands, and providing long-term service to customers after their purchases. Social aspects include recognizing employees for their accomplishments, participating in celebratory events such as the births of grandchildren and holiday parties, and making sure that employees bring a positive attitude toward their workday given the contributions they know they can make. Other terms management theorists use include *technical* for the task aspects of a job, and *human relations* for the social aspects.

These two aspects of leadership deserve the same amount of attention. If managers emphasize only the social aspects, they are engaging in *country club leadership*. The workplace may be pleasant and people may have a good time, but the goals of the company to provide high-quality products at a fair price and to ensure customer service receive insufficient attention (Greenberg & Baron, 2008). The result can be bankruptcy, where both managers and employees have to search for new jobs.

If managers emphasize only the task aspects, they may pay the price of extensive employee turnover. Task-oriented managers may run a productive "tight ship," but employees may feel that they will find more job satisfaction with another employer. Ironically, they may be able to sell the job skills they developed under the task-oriented leader. Executives in other companies may know the leader's reputation and say, "If these job candidates lasted two years with that martinet, they are certain to know the technical aspects of jobs in this industry." The executives participating in the hiring process will probably know of the high turnover that the intense task leader encourages and will not label job candidates as aimless job hoppers.

Balancing the task and social aspects of life is part of American culture, even if people don't use the terms frequently. Newspaper articles often report on the superior academic performance, especially in mathematics, of elementary and high school students in Japan, Korea, Sweden, and other industrialized nations. The United States does not always fare well in these comparisons. But few American parents become noticeably upset and complain vociferously to school boards. A major reason is that parents are interested in a balance between schoolwork and the development of social skills. They want a challenging school curriculum where students learn mathematics, science, and English (task aspects), but they also want extracurricular activities where students can develop human relations skills. Parents also want their children to have time to pursue hobbies and to obtain work experience in part-time or summer jobs. Parents know that companies want their new hires to have a combination of task and social skills. They look to the American school system to help in the development of this balance.

Let's examine a critical incident involving the distinction between the task and social aspects of leadership and how inattention to one aspect can affect a person's career aspirations.

The Needs of People and the Expectations of Task Accomplishment: Finding a Balance

The senior executives of a large computer manufacturing company met to decide on promotions. There was one opening for a division manager, and a number of well-qualified people had applied. One person, Mike Iwamoto, was an "in-house" candidate, having worked in the company for eight years.

Mike's yearly evaluations emphasized that the technical aspects of his programming skills were excellent, and that he always delivered his work on time. He wrote good reports about his work so that senior executives knew of his contributions. His written suggestions about marketing to colleges and universities through stores that sold textbooks had resulted in increased sales. People on the promotion committee who knew Mike agreed that the yearly evaluations were accurate and summarized his reputation in the company. Despite these positive aspects of his past work, Mike was passed over for promotion.

One reason for this negative decision was that Mike had not balanced task and social aspects in the workplace. There are many theories concerning what makes a good manager or a good leader, and there are several concepts that are central to all of them.

In all theories, an essential element to people moving up the ladder in an organization is the combination of skills at the technical aspects of their jobs (task) with competence in human relations skills (social). Mike's evaluations emphasized the task aspects of his work: computer programming, meeting deadlines, report writing, and insights into potential new markets. But there was nothing mentioned about various social skills. Does Mike work well with others? Is he willing to share his programming expertise with colleagues? Is he a pleasant coworker who contributes to a positive work environment? Without a reputation for competence in these areas, people are often passed over for promotion despite considerable technical skills.

Some social skills might not be reflected in a yearly performance review, but they are still important in developing and maintaining a positive reputation in one's workplace. People should be willing to stop and chat with others, especially during breaks and lunch hours. They should do their share of "oohing and aahing" when shown new pictures of a coworker's grandchildren. They should bring their share of food to company potluck parties. In Hawaii, they must give a gift if invited to the high school graduation of a colleague's son or daughter. Participation in these activities helps a person develop a reputation as "approachable." At coffee breaks and company potlucks people inevitably "talk shop" and exchange information about projects and developments in their areas of expertise. With knowledge about a person's approachability and technical expertise, others might then contact the person when they need help with an aspect of their work. This willingness to share contributes to the person's reputation as a cooperative colleague, and it keeps the person in the pool of workers who will be considered for promotion.

DESIRABLE QUALITIES POSSESSED BY LEADERS

In an extensive study carried out in 60 countries, Robert House and his colleagues (2004) identified a universal preference that employees have for their leaders. This quality is an aspect of the complex term *charisma*. Employees prefer leaders who have the ability to communicate a clear vision of the future and to communicate how employees can contribute to this vision. If they accept the vision, employees are convinced that both they and the company will prosper. Employees don't always find the desirable qualities that they desire, but they keep looking and hoping.

Charisma

The ability to paint a vision of the future that is clear to employees and to other organizational stockholders (e.g., investors, customers) is part of charisma (Aycan, 2008). Successful executives are often asked about the traits of effective leaders. Along with honesty and integrity, executives often point to charisma as a desirable trait. Often, however, the term is not fully explained and so many people do not have a clear understanding of charismatic leadership.

There are three uses of the term *charisma*. The first, and probably the most common, refers to exciting personalities who seem to fill the room once they come in the door. Many charismatic leaders have the talent of making any one individual feel as if he or she is the center of the world. Further, charismatic leaders generate enthusiasm for their work, and others adopt this positive attitude. Positive attention from charismatic leaders is a reward, and so people put forth their best efforts to please the leaders.

A second type of charisma refers to leaders who are successful in communicating a vision about the future. They are successful when telling others that if they invest their resources and support the leader's vision, everyone will benefit. Charismatic leaders of this second type are not necessarily exciting and vibrant people. Instead of these qualities, they often communicate a quiet confidence about their abilities and also demonstrate competencies necessary to achieve their goals. The classic example of this type of leadership is Bill Gates. He may not have an exciting and effervescent personality, but people who invested in his early vision about the potential of personal computers are now very wealthy.

Some leaders combine these two types of charisma: they are awe-inspiring people who are "larger than life," and they communicate a clear vision of what the future holds if their leadership is accepted. My father served under General George Patton during World War II. General Patton was certainly a colorful and domineering personality, but he also could persuade others to accept his vision. He was able to communicate to soldiers that if they followed him, they would return to their families as victors.

A third type of charisma refers to leaders who are very successful at meeting expectations of followers. In a nonprofit organization, people often feel that leaders should be good public speakers, should have many community contacts, and be good at fund-raising. If leaders meet these expectations through effective work in their day-to-day behaviors, then they possess this third type of charisma. Different cultures have different expectations of leaders (Aycan, 2008; Smith, 2008), and so a charismatic leader in one country may not have this reputation in another. In many Asian countries, leaders are expected to be very paternalistic and to take a personal interest in the lives of their employees. For example, if employees are unmarried, leaders can introduce people to potential romantic partners. This happens infrequently in the United States where expectations about leaders do not include this level of involvement in employees' personal lives.

Ability to Establish and Communicate Organizational Culture

Like charisma, *culture* is a complex term that needs explanation. My students often comment, "You tell us about cultural differences between people who have recently moved to Hawaii and people who have lived here all their lives (Brislin, 2008). We have also heard the term *organizational culture* used when referring to different companies in different parts of the world. Is the term *culture* being used in the same way?"

Culture refers to shared attitudes, values, and behaviors that are familiar to people who live in the same community and who speak the same language (Brislin, 2000). When applied to organizations, the use of the term *culture* is similar. Organizations have norms that guide behavior, and people who work for the same company often have similar attitudes toward key business issues such as ethics, customer service, and participative decision making. When studying a society's culture, a key issue is that attitudes and values are passed from generation to generation. Young adults see their culture in the behavior of their parents and grandparents.

With organizations, there is also transfer of information and values from older to younger people, but the number of years per "generation" is shorter. With organizational culture, the length of a generation is the average number of years people spend in a company. For fast food restaurants, a generation is short, perhaps no more than a year. For a well-established bank, the typical tenure of employees is much longer and consequently generations are marked by larger number of years.

Knowledge of organizational culture allows people to answer the question, "What sort of place is this to work over a long period of time?" Organizational culture (Erez & Shokef, 2008) is summarized in the stories people tell generation after generation. In a large office supply store for which I consulted, the owner's 25-year-old son returned home after earning his MBA degree at a prestigious university. Expecting an executive position, he asked his father, "What job do you want me to take on?" His father handed him a mop and broom and pointed to an area that needed cleaning. This story was told over and over in the company to communicate an important part of the organization's culture. Everyone in the company starts at the bottom and works their way up based on proven abilities. This aspect of culture was clearly communicated by the organization's leader.

Other aspects of organizational culture are summarized in images of the heroes and heroines in the organization. Who opened up new niche markets for the company? Who rose to the level of vice president even though he didn't have a college degree? Who should we look to for guidance when we want to improve our customer service? Heroes and heroines embody traits and behaviors of an organization's most valued employees. These people are often kept in mind as summarizing the standards to be met when companies interview candidates for new hires. If candidates know why certain people are considered heroes and heroines, they have an advantage during the interview process.

DEVELOPING LEADERSHIP QUALITIES

As previously mentioned, there is no dearth of advice on how to become a leader (Yukl, 2010). I regularly teach a course in leadership to college juniors and seniors, have introduced and administered complex programs in organizations, and have had formal leadership titles. I frequently ask people who have read a reasonable number of books and research articles on leadership and whom I respect in their own day-to-day work, "What advice would you give me, or any person accepting a leadership position?" Four of the answers they give center on accepting disagreements, developing trusting relationships (Fukuyama, 1995), communicating a positive attitude and a sense of optimism, and modeling and encouraging organizational citizenship. Each of these will now be discussed.

Accepting Disagreements

There are often distinctions that executives make when discussing the university graduates whom they might hire. The executives often respond by starting with skills with which they are pleased. These include technical abilities such as computer literacy, accounting, statistics, and forecasting. They would like to see more emphasis placed on writing skills, oral communication, and the ability to work cooperatively in groups. What do these desired skills have in common?

In business school jargon, executives want to see job applicants who have evidence of "soft or people skills," "the soft side of organizations," and "human relations emphases." The element that all the desired qualities have in common is that people must present their ideas to others and then receive feedback. People must present their potential contributions in written or oral form. These contributions can be formal or informal. Business plans are very formal documents and are essential to attract interest in new projects. Informal notes in the form of memos and e-mails keep others up-to-date on developments in the organization. Hour-long presentations to an organization's highest level executives can take weeks to prepare. Making suggestions to others in informal meetings is important in the development and maintenance of positive group efforts in the workplace.

After any of these written or oral presentations, people receive feedback. In the hour-long presentation, they will know whether or not they have kept the attention of the company's executives by reading their audience's nonverbal reactions. They may be told "good work" after both written and oral submissions. In the more informal give-and-take of contributions during group meetings, they may find that others disagree with their ideas. The ability to keep up positive relations with people who frequently disagree is an extremely important part of job success and career development.

Many people find it very difficult to interact with people who disagree with them (Brislin, 2008). These people attribute disagreement as a challenge to their worth as individuals. Occasionally, disagreement becomes genuine criticism, as when a boss points out that a person was careless during the preparation of an oral or written presentation. People must learn to accept such criticism with graciousness and to use it to improve their next presentation.

The fear of disagreement and criticism frequently motivates people to avoid making presentations and to keep silent during meetings with workgroup members. The inability to disagree and to benefit from criticism will have an impact on performance during job interviews and during the early years of career development. During interviews, some panel members will ask what people will do if they find themselves in frequent disagreements with coworkers. Or, panel members will disagree with something job applicants say just to gauge their reactions.

Business school faculty members have responded to the desires of executives. Students give oral presentations in class to their peers. One student told me this semester, "I have an oral presentation in each of the four classes I am taking." They also write extensively and are given feedback on both the quality of their ideas and their styles of presentation. I also advise students to join groups where other members will probably disagree with them on a variety of issues. If they join the finance committee of any club, for example, I guarantee there will be disagreements about how club dues will be spent. If people can "thicken up their skins" and learn to disagree in a constructive manner, they will have a talent that will serve them well in their workplaces.

Developing Trusting Relationships

Success in the workplace demands the involvement of other people. Leaders and people with leadership aspirations must develop relations with others that involve cooperation and trust (Fukuyama, 1995). One reason is that jobs have become so complex, especially in their technical demands, that everyone can benefit from both receiving and offering assistance. Typical questions cooperative people ask each other include, "Do you know more about this new software than I do? Who would be a good lawyer to include in these negotiations? Do you know a financial adviser who could help me with investments?"

If people develop close relationships with others, they must learn to trust one another. Trust always involves vulnerability. Others may take advantage of what were thought to be trusting relationships. Vulnerability can involve many issues. If people are cheated in financial transactions by colleagues they trusted, they are likely to become extremely upset. Trust can also be broken when people feel that confidential information has been leaked to an organization's competitors. Working with outsiders to their company, two engineers may have shared information about company secrets concerning new technologies. They trusted that the outsiders would consider the information both confidential and proprietary. If the outsiders share this information with the company's competitors, the engineers will become known as careless and as poor judges of character. This will affect their reputations, and they may find that they are not asked to become involved in sensitive projects. Lack of such invitations to become involved in important projects will lead to career stagnation.

Another type of vulnerability involves personal information that people do not want widely divulged. If two individuals develop a close relationship, there is almost always highly personal information that they share with one another. This information can include past relationships that went sour, what they really think about their boss, difficulties with their children, and what their personal long-term goals are. When people who were once close friends cease their relationship, a reason for their parting often involves the violation of trust concerning such confidential information. One individual thought that a piece of highly personal information would not be shared outside the friendship. The other person blabbed the information to others. People take these violations very seriously and do not forget them quickly.

When people move from place to place, it is wise to be attentive to norms concerning when people communicate information to others (Brislin, 2008; Hall, 1959; 1966). Difficulties arise when one person feels that personal information should remain confidential, but the other does not receive this message. Assume a person tells a colleague about a negative experience in the local community. Where I was socialized (New England), a colleague would not share this information with others unless the person had specifically said that it would be acceptable to do so. In Hawaii, my observation is that people share information unless there is a specific agreement that it not be communicated with others. The "default option" is different. In one place, it is "when in doubt, don't tell others." In the other, it is "tell others unless there was an agreement not to do so." There can be misunderstandings, sometimes bitter, if people are unaware of this difference.

Developing a Positive and Optimistic Attitude

People want an organizational culture that includes the expectation that workers have positive attitudes toward themselves, coworkers, customers, and other stakeholders (Diener & Diener, 1996; Diener & Seligman, 2004; Fredrickson, 1998). Leaders need to be models of a positive outlook and optimism. In the movie, *O Brother, Where Art Thou?* the Whites sang the country music standard, "Keep on the Sunny Side of Life." the pop song from 1928, somewhat old-fashioned by today's musical tastes, advised people to "Let a Smile Be Your Umbrella." Dale Carnegie's guidance on *How to Win Friends and Influence People* emphasized the value of a positive attitude concerning interactions with others (Carnegie, 1981). Mothers tell their children, "If you can't say anything nice, don't say it!" Although the importance of positive thoughts and emotions has long been recognized, recent research in the social and behavioral sciences has documented the many benefits of optimism and cordial relationships.

Barbara Fredrickson (1998; Fredrickson & Losada, 2005) has studied the relationship between positive and negative emotions. There are benefits to positive thoughts, attitudes, and communications that go beyond the immediate good feelings that cheerfulness brings. If people display a positive attitude, they attract others who can offer various types of social resources. These include companionship, social support during times of stress, and information ("For heaven's sakes, which Medicare drug plan best applies to my needs?"). Positive emotions also encourage exploratory behaviors, and during such behaviors people may reap various benefits. If people feel good, for example, they are more likely to take a risk and visit a new and unfamiliar museum about which they recently read. At the museum they may learn something new from the exhibits, may see an old friend whom they haven't seen in a long time, and will have their natural feelings of curiosity reinforced.

If people display negative attitudes, they will not be attractive to others. Rather, others will avoid pessimistic individuals because they do not want to be dragged down into a depressing whirlpool of whining and complaining. Negativity discourages the type of exploratory behavior that places people into situations that might raise their spirits. In the absence of movement away from their current pessimistic environment, people are likely to wallow in cynicism and feelings of boredom. Finally, if people have negative views about the world, the absence of optimistic friends and pleasant exploratory experiences will not give them opportunities to correct or to modify their pessimism.

Of course, a constant display of positive emotions and behaviors is impossible. Everyone has negative experiences and thoughts given the complexity and challenges of day-to-day life. The skill that optimistic people possess is emphasizing the positive, finding value in negative experiences ("every cloud has a silver lining"), and seeking out pleasurable activities if they feel sad and blue. In people's everyday lives, there should be a greater number of positive than negative experiences. Negative experiences have more impact on people's overall sense of well-being than do positive experiences.

Readers might want to join me in some self-exploration of our interactions with others. Think of individuals we have known for a long time. Consider the positive interactions with these people. Then, consider the negative experiences that had unpleasant outcomes. Are the negative experiences more memorable and did they lead to more intense emotions? Did it take a large number of positive experiences to overcome problems brought on by the unpleasant encounters (Bandura, 2001; Peterson & Wood, 2008)? After such considerations, most people conclude that positive experiences have to outnumber the negative for friendships to continue.

Recent research suggests that people should maintain a ratio of three positive for each negative emotion over a long time period such as a month. With this ratio, the advantages of a sunny and optimistic outlook on life are available to people. If they recognize the importance of more positive than negative experiences, they can actively seek out pleasurable events should they encounter some of the inevitable bumps in the road that life will always offer.

Perhaps a few personal remarks will be helpful in this discussion of positive attitudes, optimism, and enthusiastic attitudes in the workplace. When I am not spending time with other professors, students, and businesspeople, I play music and play bridge in club and regional tournaments. As part of my community volunteer activities, I have participated in the selection of musicians for concerts that involve reasonable compensation. (I have not found a group that wants to pay to watch bridge players.) People I play music with sometimes ask me about using their musical skills to either work full time or to supplement their incomes. Their interest stimulated me to investigate the question, "Are there good musicians who have a difficult time earning money with their talent?" I believe that the answer is yes, and there are identifiable reasons for their difficulties. One problem is that some people do not realize that they must move from being musicians to being entertainers.

Good entertainers create a sense of a special time and place and are enthusiastic about their music. They create the feeling that "this is the most important concert and time with people that I have ever experienced." Let's use the example of an acoustic guitarist who plays large numbers of Hawaiian songs. Even if the guitarist has played "Pearly Shells" or "The Hawaiian Wedding Song" 1,000 times, audience members never think about this possibility. They listen to the music as if the performer is playing it for the first time in a public setting. Good musicians who lack the skill of entertaining may play a piece flawlessly but not generate excitement among audience members if the sense of "specialness" is lacking.

Another reason for the need of a special time is that musicians are not competing for audience members' leisure time guitar dollar, traditional music dollar, or even acoustic music dollar. They are competing for people's entertainment dollar and they must move beyond aficionados interested in a specialized genre of music. Entertainers know that people could be spending their leisure time money on a movie, play, symphonic concert, evening out in a restaurant, and so forth. This is the dollar that musicians are competing for, and they must find a way to communicate with people who don't know much about guitar music and who know nothing about Hawaiian music.

Musicians should communicate a sense that they are the sorts of people who would be great guests in an audience member's home. Acoustic guitarists will not regularly perform in auditoriums that seat 1,000 or more. They are more likely to find audiences in places that seat 300 or less. Musicians, then, need to create a sense of intimacy and a sense of two-way communication with the audience. Some musicians do this by telling interesting stories about specific songs and tunes. They tell where they learned the song, who taught it to them, who wrote it, what historical events were happening when the song was written, and so forth.

These guidelines concerning enthusiasm, a special time, knowing the competition, and two-way communication are useful in many different workplaces. People making sales calls, for instance, do not show boredom with potential customers just because they are pitching a product for the thousandth time. Successful salespeople treat customers as special individuals, just as successful entertainers behave toward their audiences.

Encouraging Organizational Citizenship

Some workers go beyond their job descriptions and formal expectations for their positions in their companies (Borman, 2004; Coleman & Borman, 2000; Farh, Hackett, & Chen, 2008). If they engage in such behaviors on a regular basis, they are said to engage in organizational citizenship. A company's leaders should model and encourage these helpful behaviors and should communicate to subordinates that organizational citizenship actions will pay benefits in the long run. Here is a critical incident dealing with this aspect of the workplace.

Organizational Citizenship Contributes to Career Success

Comparing himself to others at his workplace, Jim Reynolds felt that he was ready for a promotion. In his position as a software development specialist for a company that produced home entertainment products, Jim had designed two computer games that had sold well. In addition, he had successfully followed through on his supervisor's directive to prepare the technical manuals for three other programs that his company had developed. Jim felt that this record of achievement should lead to a promotion and he made an appointment with his supervisor to discuss the issue. The supervisor, however, had recently thought about whom he would recommend for promotions and decided not to support Jim. Feeling that his work was better than the supervisor's preferred candidates, Jim was extremely disappointed.

Jim's supervisor may be considering organizational citizenship behaviors in his thinking about promotions. These types of behaviors, highly valued by bosses, are those that contribute to the accomplishment of an organization's goals but that are not part of an employee's technical performance on assigned tasks. Examples of organizational citizenship include helping others, informing others of events that they do not know about, representing the organization through volunteer community activities, and going beyond the duties listed in one's job description if the organization is faced with difficult challenges. Research (Borman, 2004; Coleman & Borman, 2000) indicates that supervisors consider both technical efficiency and organizational citizenship when carrying out performance evaluations and making promotion decisions.

In his own thinking about his work, Jim had emphasized his technical skills and task productivity but did not consider his organizational citizenship (Borman, 2004). Jim is not alone. Many workers put so much emphasis on completing tasks assigned to them that they ignore other needs in the organization that are not mentioned in their formal job descriptions. In addition to maintaining technical expertise, do they contribute to such necessary tasks as mentoring new employees, making themselves available to share their expertise with coworkers, and making thoughtful and tactful suggestions concerning how the organization can be improved?

There are three types of organizational citizenship. The first type, positive interpersonal relationships in the workplace, includes helping out others with their tasks and putting team objectives ahead of personal interests. The second type, organizational support, includes promotion of the organization through community activities and participation in professional associations. The third type, showing initiative, includes persisting on tasks with extra effort despite difficult conditions, and doing so with a minimum of whining. It also includes expanding the skills that can be applied in the workplace through taking advantage of educational opportunities inside and outside of the organization.

People who increase their organizational citizenship behaviors reap benefits over and above workplace promotions. As companies strive to be more efficient, or "leaner and meaner," executives are asking employees to handle more and more tasks. Employees who have limited areas of technical expertise risk being downsized. Workers who engage in good citizenship behaviors often develop new areas of expertise because they are interacting frequently with coworkers and are attending professional conferences. Through such interactions, they become more flexible and adaptable because they are combining their skills and knowledge with the contributions of others. Combined with their willingness to show initiative, they become the types of employees that executives want to keep in their organizations and to put on their lists of people being considered for leadership roles in the future.

WHEN POTENTIAL LEADERS BECOME DERAILED

In any discussion of how people who aspire to leadership positions can develop the necessary skills, there should also be a discussion of how some people go wrong.

Becoming Derailed. At recent meetings of the Academy of Management, Robie, Brown, and Bly (2008) reported the results of research on how potentially successful managers become derailed from first-rate careers. In many companies, high-level executives identify potential "fast trackers" and give them opportunities to demonstrate their talents. The young managers are put in charge of departments or are given leadership assignments on important group tasks. Some of the managers do well and rise up through an organization's hierarchy and reach the executive ranks. Other managers do not do well. They make mistakes and are eventually derailed from successful advancement in their organizations. They become stuck in low-level managerial jobs or leave the organization with a reputation for being unsuccessful.

What is the difference between the two groups of young managers? Research suggests that the unsuccessful managers engage in behaviors that, over a long period of time, irritate so many subordinates that complaints mount and tasks are not accomplished in a timely manner. There are five types of derailing behaviors.

1. Unsuccessful managers are so ego-centered that they focus on themselves, not on the needs of their subordinates. Further, they behave in ways that suit themselves and do not keep organizational goals in mind.
2. They are intimidating, forcing compliant behaviors from subordinates rather than engaging them in collaborative efforts aimed at commonly shared goals. Subordinates may seem to go along with the managers, but they do this only when their bosses are present.
3. Unsuccessful managers are manipulative. For example, they engage in behind-the-scenes behaviors such as gossip mongering and backstabbing.
4. They are also micromanagers and do not give their subordinates credit for having the ability to carry out assigned tasks. As part of this problem, they are poor at assessing the talents of their subordinates and arranging for training programs to bring the talent level up to a point where tasks can be accomplished.
5. Finally, the unsuccessful managers are passive-aggressive when faced with people who disagree with them or who show signs of independence. This means that they will act in a positive and seemingly pleasant way during face-to-face interactions with others, but they will find opportunities to inflict revenge at a later time.

So far, the research paints a story with which many readers will be familiar given the poor bosses for whom they have worked. But there is a plot twist! For the first few years of their career development, young managers with these derailing traits are rated highly by executives! Why is this the case? At the Academy of Management meetings, participants suggested three reasons. One reason for high ratings is that executives may observe the young managers and conclude that they are very busy. If they are micromanaging and concerned with their self-image, they may come across as hardworking and dedicated people.

Another reason is that there is a sharp distinction between successful and effective. People can be rated as successful if they fit the image of industrious managers, but they may not be effective in helping the company reach goals such as new product development and market expansion. Finally, some executives like to have manipulative and passive-aggressive managers in their companies since the executives can use them to do their dirty work. Examples include introducing unpopular policies and firing workers who are well liked by colleagues.

The micromanaging and intimidating young managers eventually pay a price for their behaviors. After a few years, executives discover that the managers are not effective, breed ill will in the organization, and so the executives discontinue their support. The managers receive the outcomes they deserve: They become derailed.

Lack of Self-Insight. Leaders need to be able to ask and answer questions such as: "How am I coming across to others? If I had just received the directive that I recently circulated, how would I feel? Could I be working toward company goals in a more effective manner? Am I balancing the task and the social requirements of my leadership role?" If they can answer such questions in ways similar to that of their subordinates, leaders are said to have self-insight (London, 2001). This discussion allows me to draw from a quite different interest that I have, and I hope that readers will indulge me.

I am ready to make a confession. One of my guilty pleasures is watching "The Apprentice" on television. Various businesspeople, many of them with advanced degrees and good work experience, vie for the attentions of Donald Trump. Participants on the show break into teams and engage in various business tasks. Examples are designing a marketing plan for a new car, creating and selling a new brand of ice cream, and redesigning and renting apartments. Each week, one person performs worse than others and is fired.

I enjoy the show because the participants have to draw on their knowledge of various managerial practices. These include planning, organizing teams, motivating workers, communicating with others, leading, maintaining group morale during stressful periods, and predicting the reactions of consumers to new products. When selecting candidates for the show, I suspect that the producers choose people who are highly competent but whose personalities might clash with others. The producers know that scenes of people arguing and scheming against each other contribute to the probability of a successful program. Viewers would rather see interpersonal clashes and intrigue than see a group of highly cooperative people who show respect for each other.

There are two types of especially interesting candidates. One group is populated by people with an edge to their personalities. These people have traits that irritate others. Examples are that they talk too much, have a snarl in their voice when addressing others, think that they are smarter than everybody else, or are overly bossy when they become team leaders. Another group is composed of people who have very little self-insight. When they behave, they have no idea of how they are coming across to others. They have no ability to put themselves into the shoes of observers. They cannot examine their own behavior and predict its impact on other people.

These candidates are often among the first to get fired. One woman had a very bossy personality (House, Hanges, Javidan, Dorfman, & Gupta, 2004) but had no awareness of this fact. She told Donald Trump that she did not get along with other women because she was so beautiful. On another episode, a man chewed tobacco but was unable to understand that this habit could have an impact when he was interacting with children who were test-marketing a game that his team designed.

When producers choose candidates who show little self-insight, they cannot predict the exact types of spats they will have. They can predict, though, that they will have interesting clashes with other candidates who are highly competitive and highly confident about their abilities. A metaphor may be helpful. If people toss gasoline into a room and then throw a match, they can't predict the exact extent of the fire. They can predict, however, that some kind of fire will occur.

Self-insight is a valuable trait for leaders (London, 2001). If they decide to behave in certain ways, they are skillful at predicting how others will react. They can answer questions such as the following: "How do I come across to subordinates when I give them suggestions about their work? How would I feel if a boss gave me suggestions in the same way? Can I put myself in the shoes of my subordinates and predict their reactions to my directives given their level of job experience? Is there anything I can change about myself so that I can become a more effective manager and leader?" They can then take the answers to these self-directed questions and change their behavior so that they communicate more effectively with others.

Robert Burns (see Henley, 1897) once wrote about the value of increased self-insight: "O would some power the giftie gie us to see ourselves as others see us." While the presence of such a gift is of value to managers and leaders, its absence contributes to colorful episodes on reality television programs. Self-insight is one result of careful thinking. Such effective and efficient thinking is aided if people are aware of how the mind works, or in slightly more technical terms, how people form, deal with, and possibly benefit from their cognitions—the topic of the next chapter.

3

People's Cognitions

When young managers do not live up to their promise, senior executives in an organization often have conversations concerning why their subordinates did not perform as expected. Often, the executives' conversations consist of statements such as, "they do not think clearly," "they are unrealistic about their expectations," or "they don't encourage positive thinking in this organization." All of these statements deal with how people think, or in the slightly more technical language of experimental and social psychology, their cognitions (Bandura, 2001; Hodgkinson & Healey, 2008; Peterson & Wood, 2008).

The ability to think about the past, present, and future is unique to humans and distinguishes us from our close relatives such as the chimpanzees, bonobos, orangutans, and gorillas. There is no evidence that these other primates can think about what they might do in a few years, and no evidence that they can think about abstract thoughts such as, "How can we improve our current state of affairs to have a better life for our children?" Human beings can engage in such thoughts. The ability to think, or to have complex cognitions, also differentiates us from possible predators. We are not as fast as gazelles or horses, not as strong as lions or tigers, and cannot fly without mechanical aids and so have a disadvantage to birds. But we can think. We can develop complex weapons to hunt gazelles for food. We can build protections against stronger animals. And (more recently in our history) we can use our thinking to build machines that fly faster and farther than the strongest birds. There is some evidence that language, which allows us to express our thoughts to others, developed so that we could be more efficient in our thinking and could benefit from reactions to our ideas from others (Goldin-Meadow, 2006; Pinker, 2002).

Cognitions, and languages to express them to others, provided humans with a major advantage in the struggle for survival during the thousands of years of prerecorded history. People could say to each other, "The area where we are living now seems to have run out of food supplies. We should move, and we should move to the area in the direction of the sun, where we found food before." Or, on a specific quest for food, one person could direct others to make noise and to drive game to the hunters who were most skillful with the use of handmade spears.

The ability to think about the past, present, and future continues to mark people who are nurtured into, and who accept, leadership positions. These people are intelligent (Schmidt & Hunter, 2004), and their thinking is complex. As discussed in Chapter 2, they have self-insight, which can also be called accurate cognitions about the self. They can plan for the future, asking and answering such questions as, "What are we doing well now in this organization, and what can we be doing better? What is our competition doing? Should we do what they are doing, or should we do something else so that we differentiate ourselves from them so that we call more attention to ourselves?"

The ability to think clearly is also a benefit when analyzing potential problems. Sometimes, the issue is not what seems to be a problem, but how people are thinking about it (Moore, 2000). Cognitions, then, can be added to the analysis of problems and thus sometimes bring a sense of control to life's difficulties. Franklin Roosevelt knew this when he said, during the Depression, "We have nothing to fear but fear itself." He knew the Depression was causing severe problems, but he did not want the problems exacerbated by people's thinking that would focus solely on fear, despondency, and the belief that things will not get better. Instead, Roosevelt urged people to keep a positive outlook and to believe that improvements are in store in the future.

The importance of adding cognitions to the analysis of problems has become a contribution of psychological research that has been widely accepted among laypeople.

The message is, "Sometimes it is not what the problem appears to be, but how people think about it." For example, members of 12-step programs have the goal of staying sober. This is a challenge but it is aided by the cognitions, "My goal is to stay sober one day at a time, and I can call my sponsor if I feel I am backsliding." Addressing the big problem, sobriety, is aided by the manageable cognition dealing with one day, then another day, then another. When students come to me with the temptation to drop out of college, I sometimes say, "Can we agree that you will give college one more semester? And let's talk about your interests, and what activities you enjoy in the classroom, to see if we can identity a set of courses that will be appealing to you." The big problem, staying in school, is aided by the more manageable cognitions of "one more semester" and "courses that appeal to me, personally."

STRESS AND COGNITIONS

The fact that many people are giving attention to cognitions in the analysis of big problems became especially clear recently in a hospital-run seminar that I attended. I had an operation a few years ago, and as part of my recovery my surgeon recommended a seminar series on healthy lifestyles. Some behavior change, he suggested, would speed recovery and would contribute to long-term health with less probability of difficulties in the future. So I went to a seminar that dealt with issues such as healthy eating, exercise, and stress management. During one of the seminars on stress, the leader urged us to identity stressors in our lives, reminding us that what is stressful for one person (e.g., public speaking, playing music in public) is not stressful for another. I remember commenting, "But some of us have problems that are inherently stressful and can't be avoided. For example, we have to choose one person from five for a promotion, which means that we have to tell four people that they were not promoted. This is stressful!" The leader responded, "Many times, the potential stressor can be lessened depending on your thoughts surrounding an event such as telling people that they will not be promoted."

We then went on to discuss cognitions that would reduce stress. Knowing that the four people not promoted will want to hear about what they have done well, we can start a meeting with positive statements about their work. Then, we discuss how they can improve so that they fare better in the next round of promotions. We can make recommendations concerning activities in which they might become engaged so that they increase their skills. A potentially stressful meeting can be turned into more positive planning for the future. Although not totally eliminating the stress that accompanies the act of passing on bad news, the ability to focus on positive thinking and future improvements should decrease the stress that people experience (Daniels, Hartley, & Travers, 2006; Lazarus & Folkman, 1984).

Interactions with Others, and Life Events. There is no accident in the fact that my example of stress deals with interactions among several people. Many of life's stresses involve people's relations with others. Social scientists interested in the effects of stress on health have developed various measuring instruments. One of the best known is based on people's ratings of life events that they feel are stressful (Holmes & Rahe, 1967; Tausig, 1982). In developing the scale, researchers presented people with a known event that is highly stressful for almost everyone. This event, known as an anchor, is the death of a spouse when a couple had a loving and highly committed relationship. This event is given a score of 100. Then, people consider other events and tell how stressful they are while keeping this anchor in mind.

Some stressful behaviors involve their places of employment. Being fired yields a stress score of 47 points. This score is undoubtedly higher if people face a tight job market where employers have many applicants competing for available jobs. Adjusting to a major workplace disruption brought on by changing economic conditions has a stress score of 39 points. Having trouble with one's boss brings a score of 23 points. If people have two or three bosses and are having difficulties with all of them, then this score is doubled or tripled. People might be able to cope with one troublesome relationship involving their boss, but two or three hassles can add up to a stress level that threatens their health.

Several behaviors receive stress ratings that may seem surprisingly high. Experiencing an outstanding personal achievement receives a stress score of 28 points. Why is this stressful? Wouldn't people think that personal achievements are pleasurable and could actually counteract other ongoing stresses in their lives? One reason is that if an achievement is outstanding, there is usually a ceremony and publicity attached to it. The person receiving the achievement may receive congratulations from many well-wishers at the same moment. Thanking each individual personally, showing appreciation graciously, and not shortchanging anyone by giving them too little attention can challenge a person's social skills. It would be easy to suggest that people should practice being gracious with multiple well-wishers. But even the most able people receive only one or a few major awards during their lifetimes and so practice is difficult.

Another reason personal achievements bring stress is that others may expect the person to keep up the same level of productivity and to win similar awards in the future. Again, social skills have to be very well-developed if a person can gently remind others that award-winning performances cannot be expected every day.

Experiencing activities during the Christmas season can bring a stress score of 12 points (Holmes & Rahe, 1967). One reason is that if people are coping with other troubles in their lives, seeing coworkers joyfully participating in various Christmas events can intensify their own feelings of sadness or loneliness. Mildly troubled people may try to be good employees and sing the Christmas songs during office parties and applaud when Santa enters the door. However, these appeals to their social skills can be stressful since they have to put energy into masking their true thoughts and feelings in the presence of others.

Cognitions Surrounding Stress. Different people react in various ways to potential sources of stress in the workplace, and these differences are often due to people's cognitions surrounding potentially stressful events (Daniels et al., 2006; Lazarus & Folkman, 1984).

Imagine two people who work in the same high-pressure office marked by fast-moving technological changes, unpredictable markets, demanding customers, and intense bosses who pounce on the slightest error. One person remains calm and in control and even seems to thrive on pressure. The other becomes noticeably upset. His blood pressure and heart rate increase, he approaches problems with the attitude that he can't do anything about them, and he is less effective in the everyday performance of his job duties. In short, he is "stressed out." What are the differences between the two people?

I have found a three-stage model of workplace stress to be very helpful (Lazarus & Folkman, 1984). In the first stage, people assess whether a potential stressor might affect their behavior. For some people, speaking in public is a stressor, but others are very comfortable with this task. For some customer service representatives, dealing with angry and shouting clients is very disconcerting. On the other hand, some representatives look on these clients as a challenge and enjoy calming them down so that issues can be effectively addressed. The question people can ask, then, is whether or not a potential source of stress is a concern for them.

If people feel that a stressor may lead to difficulties, they enter the second stage. Here, they assess whether they have various resources that will allow them to cope effectively. Resources include knowledge and experience. If people are asked to speak in public, stress is reduced if they have taken courses in public speaking and can choose the topic. A major source of resources for coping is a person's support group. Different people can offer various kinds of help: emotional uplifts, key information, and volunteered time to help meet an approaching deadline.

If people assess their coping resources and still feel overwhelmed, they can enter the third stage, known as *benign reappraisal*. This term refers to thought processes that lead people to put their stress in a proper perspective. They can ask themselves, "Is this problem so overwhelming that I should allow myself to become so stressed as to affect my health? Can I break down this seemingly complex problem into a series of steps that I can manage? Are there larger issues than this potential stressor, such as the well-being of my family, that I should also attend to?" With benign reappraisal, people often reduce their stress by viewing their problems as more controllable and manageable than they first thought. This approach to thinking reminds me of the serenity prayer from 12-step programs. People ask for acceptance of the things they cannot change, the courage to change the things they can, and the wisdom to know the difference.

Many stresses can be alleviated if people turn to others with whom they have well-developed relationships. These others can sometimes give helpful advice for dealing with stress and sometimes can provide emotional support. Just having someone to talk with can reduce stress and move people away from the health risks of suffering in silence.

COMPARISONS WITH OTHERS

Another important set of cognitions, also involving other people, compares what we do with what others do (Thibaut & Kelley, 1959). The others are often a collection of people with whom we have contact and look to for guidance in determining answers to the question, "Am I doing OK, or should I work on improving my life?" We can see such cognitions at work in this critical incident.

The Comparison Level of Alternatives

As roommates at Oregon State University, Mike Wilson and Brad Kim frequently talked about their futures. Both had studied business administration and had on-the-job experience through the university's internship program. Both were about to graduate and began talking about job interviews. Originally from Portland, Oregon, Mike had already participated in a number of interviews. Brad, originally from Honolulu, wanted to return home and planned most of his interviews after graduation. Brad knew about the job market through e-mail correspondence with old friends, web sites, and from the Sunday newspaper his parents sent him each week.

Comparing notes, Mike found that he was interviewing for jobs that paid as much as $10,000 a year more than jobs in Hawaii. Mike also remembered Brad's stories about coping with the cost of living in Hawaii. One day, Mike asked Brad, "How do you feel about the salary structure for jobs in Hawaii? If it bothers you, why don't you interview for some jobs here in Oregon or Washington?" Brad replied that he wanted to live in Hawaii because he valued many aspects of the culture and lifestyle: the climate, closeness to family, the soft interpersonal style among people, and year-round outdoor sports. He added, "I've long known about the salary structure for jobs in Hawaii, and people who want to live in Hawaii learn to live with it."

Mike and Brad have encountered a *different comparison level of alternatives* (Thibaut & Kelley, 1959). This term refers to decisions based on comparisons among various possibilities. The possibilities or alternatives, however, differ among various people. Rather than compare themselves with a set and unchanging standard, people make decisions based on comparisons with others who are in similar circumstances. For Mike, his comparison level will be the salaries received by Oregon State graduates who are seeking jobs in the Pacific Northwest. For Brad, his comparison level will be the salaries received by graduates from various universities who are seeking employment in Hawaii. If Brad receives similar compensation as others who are accepting jobs in Hawaii, he will be satisfied.

Even though they don't use the term, people make decisions based on comparisons between themselves and others who have similar ambitions and qualifications. People are very adept at assessing their qualifications and skills, researching the job market in cities where they want to live, and seeking matches between their skills and current job offerings. If their outcomes compare favorably to others with similar qualifications seeking jobs in the same city, they are satisfied. When they read about recent college graduates accepting salaries of $90,000 and above in New York City or Washington, D.C., they do not become disappointed or resentful. Given that they want to live in a certain place with a certain lifestyle, jobs in these big cities are not part of their comparison level of alternatives.

STEREOTYPES

One of the clearest examples of people's use of cognitions is their appeal to stereotypes (Allport, 1954; Brewer, 2007; Brislin, 2000; Risen, Gilovich, & Dunning, 2007). Most people have been the victim of stereotypes. Others put them into a category, such as Anglo male, Japanese-American, Republican, or athlete on scholarship. Then, these others use information from the stereotype in thinking about the others and making judgments (Kelley, 1967; Rousseau, 2001). When people are the targets of stereotypes, others do not make efforts to move beyond group labels and to treat people as individuals. People complain that their unique qualities are being ignored when others treat them according to some category label. Further, people may not agree that a certain imposed category label is at all applicable to them.

When I give talks in the community about workplace behavior in places where people from many cultures live (e.g., in British Columbia, California, Florida, Texas, Hawaii), issues surrounding stereotypes are frequently the topic of people's questions. Many people do not like to hear discussions of ethnic groups that are based on stereotypes. They sometimes ask me how stereotypes can be eliminated. While I agree with them about the overly frequent use of stereotypes, I have to point out that attempts to eliminate them will be like tilting at windmills.

Stereotypes are a special type of category, and people need categories to organize the thousands of specific pieces of information that they have in their memories (Kelley, 1967; Brislin, 2000). Examples of categories include edible foods, criteria of effective schools, good workplace conditions, and interesting leisure time activities. When faced with a new piece of information, people use their existing categories. If a new food resembles something that people have enjoyed in the past, they might eat it. When faced with a new job offer, they can consult their category that summarizes information and preferences concerning attractive working conditions. Using their existing categories, people do not have to do extensive thinking concerning each new piece of information. Even if people had the inclination for such careful thinking, they often do not have the time given their busy lives.

Stereotypes are categories about groups of people (Allport, 1954; Brislin, 2008). We could use the phrase "people category," but *stereotype* is a twentieth-century term that has entered the English language and that has achieved widespread use. When others meet people for the first time, they don't have to do the long-and-hard work of getting to know the people as individuals. Rather, they can assign stereotypes based on easily accessed information. People's physical appearance leads to guesses about their ethnic group. Their language use gives clues about their socioeconomic background. If they mention a few things about themselves during early encounters, such as their political affiliation, additional stereotypical information becomes available.

Stereotypes cannot be eliminated but decision making based on group characteristics and images can be countered. If people know about stereotypes, they can resist the temptation to use them when thinking about an individual whom they have just met. They can remind themselves that they should seek out information about a person's unique qualities and should not depend on facile and often erroneous generalizations.

POSITIVE AND NEGATIVE THINKING

Some people, given their genetic composition, are blessed with the tendency to engage in positive thinking about many events in their lives (Diener & Diener, 1996; Diener & Seligman, 2004; Seligman, 1991). In the words of an old song, they look at the world through rose-colored glasses, or in the words of another song, they let a smile be their umbrella. Other people have more negative thoughts and can be counted on to whine, complain, and to find fault with others. While some people may have a natural head start, everyone can make attempts to be more positive and can reap a set of benefits from so doing.

An Optimistic Thinking Style. When faced with adversity, some people react in a helpless manner and do not make attempts to overcome difficulties (Seligman, 1975). Other people react to adversity with a positive outlook, viewing difficulties as hurdles to be overcome. What is the difference between the two groups? People who bounce back from setbacks often have an optimistic thinking style (Diener & Diener, 1996; Seligman, 1991). For example, a woman may apply for a job in her community that is very attractive: excellent salary, good working conditions, and opportunities for advancement. She buys an expensive suit for the job interview. She meets members of the selection committee and has long conversations about her qualifications. But she does not get a job offer.

There are three elements in an optimistic thinking style that allow people to move forward after such disappointments (Seligman, 1991). They think about the setback in a specific rather than a general manner. *Specific* means *this* job and *this* job interview. *General* means all jobs and all interviews in the future. If people can focus on the specific setback, they will not mope about their limited chances for other good jobs. Optimistic thinkers focus on the unstable rather than the stable aspects of their job search. *Unstable* means that companies, interviewers, and job markets change, and these may change in people's favor! *Stable* means that people think that their job search failures will remain steadfastly in place no matter how hard they try to change.

The third element is that people consider external aspects of their problems and do not focus solely on internal issues. *External* refers to issues outside the control of people who are seeking jobs. One external reason for job interview disappointments is that the selection panel had a sweetheart candidate. Panel members had a person in mind all along, but went through the motions of an open search for legal reasons. Clearly, job candidates should not blame themselves if they are competing with a sweetheart. *Internal* means that people focus on themselves and their perceived shortcomings, and they often become overly harsh in their self-assessments. If they are too self-critical, they may talk themselves into inaction and not seek other good jobs.

When the external-internal distinction is discussed, I recommend that people try to maintain a balance between these two reasons for setbacks. There are often internal reasons that should be examined: interview style, questions a job candidate chooses to ask, attractiveness of resumes, and so forth. The recommended additional focus on the external factor is meant to move people away from self-blame and hopelessness for the future.

This optimistic thinking style focusing on specific issues, instability, and a balance between external and internal factors can be practiced and then applied to many problems that people face as part of their daily lives.

Drawbacks of a More Negative Thinking Style. Not everyone accepts the advice of researchers such as Seligman (1991) and instead persist in a more negative style of thinking. Some disadvantages can be seen in this incident.

Negative Expectation Can Lead to Self-Fulfilling Prophecies

The owners of a small department store in a town of 60,000 residents read that a big-box retailer, part of a national chain, would be opening a store nearby. The owners were afraid that they could not compete with a megastore and that they would go out of business. They told employees about this future competition. The department store became a gloomy place to work and customers stopped coming even before the megastore opened.

The company owners are guilty of encouraging a self-fulfilling prophecy (Merton, 1957; Sprangenberg & Scott, 2006). When people expect that something bad will happen, they begin to behave in ways that make the prophecy turn into fact. Their vision becomes self-fulfilling. The owners believed that events would occur, they behaved consistently with those prophesized events, and their actions contributed to the eventual outcome. Interactions with employees played an important role. The owners communicated their fears to employees who undoubtedly began worrying about their jobs. The employees were then likely to put time and energy into thinking about finding other jobs rather than attending to good customer service. Combined with the gloomy atmosphere at the department store, customers may have received the message that their patronage was not welcome. They stopped coming, contributing to declining sales even before the megastore was built.

Self-fulfilling prophecies can also be positive. If the department store owners communicate a sense of optimism and ask for constructive suggestions from employees, they may find that they can stay in business. The owners of small stores can identify types of customers who will not be well served by a big retail store that is part of a national chain. For example, some customers like the personal service from well-trained salespeople that megastores cannot always provide. Or, the owners may find that they can develop a loyal customer base through follow-up services after the purchase of products. The key is that an optimistic attitude may bring improvements that will allow the store to compete. A negative attitude will almost certainly lead to doom.

Self-fulfilling prophecies have effects in many aspects of life. If people over 50 years of age have a positive attitude about the future, they will engage in behaviors that will contribute to good health. They will exercise, stop smoking, be careful about their weight, and nurture close friendships. If teachers expect their students to do well, they will put time and effort into creating classroom activities that allow students to shine (Rosenthal & Jacobson, 1968).

I have long admired University of Hawaii athletic coaches who do not whine and complain about the rigors of their teams' travel to road games. The closest teams that the University of Hawaii plays are in California, approximately 2,500 miles away. It is harder to travel East from Hawaii than it is for opposing teams to travel West from the mainland. In addition, Hawaii teams have to make multiple long trips during a season although visiting teams only travel once to Hawaii. The coaches know that if they dwelt on the rigors of travel to road games, they would be communicating a negative attitude to athletes. Travel from Hawaii in the inimitable charms of coach class could become an excuse for losing. Instead coaches focus on a more positive attitude with statements such as, "All teams have to travel, good teams win on the road, and we have prepared ourselves to win."

PLANNING: COMBINING STYLES OF THINKING

I'm sure it is clear to readers that I am not recommending that people constantly engage in positive cognitions. The world is full of difficulties, and we must engage in careful thinking about negative possibilities in our lives. Once negative possibilities are identified, however, we can engage in positive planning to overcome or to lessen them.

Benjamin Franklin once wrote that there are two certainties in life: death and taxes. To these, we can add that today's complex life includes future problems for which we cannot be totally prepared. Often, the inability to deal with unforeseen problems leads to stress with negative effects on health and psychological well-being. Although life's problems and stresses cannot be reduced, people can take steps to minimize their negative impact.

When people take steps today that can reduce the impact of problems that may occur in the future, they are engaging in preventive activities. In primary prevention, people do not have certain problems today. However, they are concerned they might have the problems at a later date and so take steps to ward off future difficulties. One example is exercise. People may not have health problems today, but they realize that they may have them in the future. So they engage in an exercise program to prevent or to minimize threats to their health. Exercise helps people lose weight, and this leads to a decreased chance of adult onset diabetes; it also helps people lower their cholesterol and to keep blood pressure at a level approved by their physicians.

People can engage in primary prevention as part of their work. If they dread speaking in front of others but know that future promotions depend on the ability to give public presentations, they can sign up for seminars where they can develop this skill. Community colleges frequently offer courses in public speaking. Realizing that they will face challenges to their technical skills in the workplace, people often nurture a support group of people knowledgeable in information technology, accounting, and statistical forecasting.

If people enter into activities known as secondary prevention, they recognize that a potential stressor has entered their lives. So they take steps to minimize the negative impact of stress. If the stressor is medical, such as a pain in the abdomen or a dark blotch on their skin, they recognize the advantages of early detection and schedule a visit to their physician as soon as possible. In the workplace, people asked to give a public presentation can call on friends for various kinds of help. People might preview their talks in front of others. Or perhaps they can form a panel where a number of colleagues give parts of a full presentation. People's support groups, called on when difficulties are imminent, are often nurtured as part of primary prevention.

In tertiary prevention, people have experienced problems and stress. However, they put their experiences into perspective. They say to themselves, "Is this problem really so large that I should let it have negative impacts on my health?" Tertiary prevention also includes sorting problems into those that can be controlled and those that cannot. For problems that cannot be controlled, the advice of friends to "let it go!" is often wise. My mother captured tertiary prevention when she chided her children if they whined about a trivial issue. She advised us to "save your tears for a broken leg."

COGNITIVE ACTIVITY DOES NOT ALWAYS YIELD POSITIVE RESULTS

Although the ability to engage in complex thinking is one of the hallmarks of humans, such activity does not guarantee positive outcomes. We make mistakes. As previously discussed, we fall prey to stereotypical thinking and engage in so much negative thinking that we irritate others. If thinking were always effective, we would see happier people, better decision making, and longer-lasting interpersonal relationships. I'd like to discuss three problematic areas surrounding people's cognitive activity: difficulties with planning for the future, chasing sunk costs, and engaging in the transmission of rumors.

Thinking About the Future. People believe that they can make accurate predictions about the future, but this belief is often shattered (Hodgkinson & Healey, 2008; Kahneman, 2003). One reason is that people are poor at predicting future events that might interfere with the plans that they make today. Consider this critical incident.

Plans Concerning Future Behaviors often Go Astray

After three months on the job as president of a company that prepared and sold frozen foods, Nolan Slye called a meeting of all
300 employees. He outlined his goals for the future of the company,
which included the addition of various ethnic foods to its product line
and the expansion of markets to other countries. He promised that he
would have an open-door policy and that any employee could drop
into his office if he or she had concerns. "I believe that I can get to
know each of you personally," he continued, "and that we can all
work together to make this a place where people look forward to coming to work." He also promised that in one year, he would ask people
to participate in a 360-degree evaluation of himself. This meant that he
would seek opinions concerning his job performance from many different sources. Evaluators would include workers in the company, suppliers, customers, and homeowners who lived near the company.

Over the following year, Nolan became increasingly busy. He was asked
to become involved in various community events such as the yearly fund-
raiser for local charities. He became active in a professional organization
that dealt with food processing and accepted a position on its board of
directors. He found that he had to hire two new managers from outside
rather than from inside the company and that he was spending more time
with them than he had planned. At the end of the year, the plan for a 360-
degree evaluation was put on the back burner. Nolan did not discuss
plans for a self-evaluation at staff meetings, and no one in the company
felt comfortable enough to remind him of his promise.

Nolan has experienced a problem captured in the old adage, "The
best laid plans of mice and men often go astray." People often make
commitments that they find themselves unable to keep (Hodgkinson &
Healey, 2008; Kahneman, 2003). Everyday examples include promises
to give up smoking, to cut down on trips to Las Vegas because of gambling losses, and to be more patient with one's teenaged children. Why
do these plans go astray? One reason is the difference between verbal
statements and actual behavior.

It is much, much easier to make statements about one's future behavior than to actually carry out one's plans. Another reason is that people
are not skillful at predicting possible unforeseen events that will interfere with their verbal plans. In the case of smoking, people are rarely
able to foresee stressful events that will tempt them to search for a
pack of cigarettes. In the gambling example, people are unable to predict their reactions when they hear that their high school reunion will
be meeting in Las Vegas.

In addition to poor prediction of unforeseen events, people are also
inept at predicting their future emotions associated with their current

plans. In Nolan's case, he promised a 360-degree evaluation of himself in one year. So the year is up! Where is the evaluation? Nolan might not feel like having an evaluation of himself. After a year, there will certainly be some negative commentary, and not everyone enjoys hearing such feedback. For example, Nolan hired two outside managers. Candidates from inside the company are undoubtedly disappointed, and Nolan knows that they could use the evaluation process to vent their feelings. In addition, Nolan may have become quite comfortable with the power that accompanies his position as president of a company. He has become active in community affairs and in a national organization. He may feel that it is beneath his self-assessed dignity to seek feedback from people who have not risen to his current level in the status hierarchy (Brislin, 1991).

Chasing Sunken Costs. After people invest resources such as money, time, effort, and emotion, they do not like to admit that their resources have been wasted. This can lead to ineffective thinking known as chasing sunk costs (He & Mittal, 2007).

Chasing Sunk Costs Can Go beyond Money

Having won awards for both his short stories and essays, Jack Dodson wants to pursue a career as a professional writer. To gain experience, he spends a great deal of time writing articles for a weekly shopping market publication that consumers use to determine the stores with the best money-saving sales. Jack figures that he makes about $5 an hour for this work. But he also feels that if he writes well, other prestigious newspapers and magazines will offer him lucrative writing assignments. He continues to write for the shopping market weekly, and most of his time is taken up with this writing, his "straight job" as a security guard, and his family life. But offers for better paying writing assignments do not appear.

Jack may be making the error of chasing sunk costs. When people invest resources into products, activities, or relationships, they may later engage in behaviors meant to protect these initial investments. The clearest cases of sunk costs involve money, leading to the frequently heard advice, "Don't throw good money after bad!" Assume that a person owns a 1982 Ford Mustang and has a sentimental attachment to it since it is the car he used when courting his wife. Nine months ago he spent $900 on a brake job. Six months ago, he spent $600 on a new carburetor. Yesterday, his mechanic told him he needed a new transmission, and the costs for parts and labor would be $1,200. Should the car owner tell the mechanic to go ahead? He surely wants to say to himself, "If I invest money for this last repair, I'll have reliable transportation for years to come." But if he approves the new transmission, he may be chasing the sunk costs of the first two repairs. Perhaps he should junk the Mustang and invest the $1,200 in a new car.

Sunk costs apply to relationships. Take the example of a couple that has been dating for five years. The relationship has been rocky, as friends and family members have often observed. But the two people say to each other, "Let's give this relationship six more months to see if we can work things out!" This may be a good idea, but it also may be an example of chasing sunk costs. In this case, the "cost" is six more months to protect the investment of the previous five years.

If people recognize the possibility of sunk costs, they can examine their various investments and think carefully about which ones deserve additional resources and which do not. At times, they will conclude that they have to cut their losses, whether the loss is a poorly performing stock, a career option, or a relationship. If they do not cut their losses, they risk entering an endless cycle of throwing today's resources after yesterday's problematic decisions (He & Mittal, 2007; Johnson & Hoopes, 2003).

Engaging in Rumor Transmission. Good managers have insights into human behavior, and one insight is that they know that employees will use the great gift of being able to think (Hodgkinson & Healey, 2008). Realizing this, managers give their subordinates information so that they can think clearly. If managers do not communicate accurate information and leave subordinates wondering what is going on in the organization, there will be dangerous outcomes. One outcome is that employees will participate in the creation and dissemination of rumors (Allport & Postman, 1945; DiFonzo & Bordia, 2007).

Rumors Fly around Organizations in the Absence of Solid Information

In recent years, 30 stores in the Music Is Us chain had become established in California and Oregon. The owner of the stores, Jack Davis, wanted to appeal to amateur and professional vocalists and instrumentalists who wanted to expand their repertoires. He also had a good market among parents of school children who needed good-quality but reasonably priced ukuleles, harmonicas, and recorders for their music classes.

In the early summer of 2009, however, sales seemed to be declining. "Maybe musicians have enough materials to expand their horizons, and maybe neighbors are sharing their children's instruments with each other," Jack suggested to his management team. Looking at the performance of various stores, Jack identified three that might have to be downsized or possibly closed. Before taking such steps, however, he wanted to wait for "back to school" shoppers who might buy materials for their schoolchildren. He asked his management team to keep these plans confidential because he did not want to upset his employees. Two weeks later, Mark began to hear stories about the future of Music Is Us. The stories bore no resemblance to reality. "The rumor mills have been working overtime," he complained.

Rumors are circulated about important issues when there is an absence of solid information (Allport & Postman, 1945; DiFonzo & Bordia, 2007). Jack's first mistake was thinking that the plans for possible store closings would stay within his management team. Someone from the team will talk. One might tell a tennis-playing friend, who will then tell a neighbor. The neighbor, shopping at a Music Is Us store, will mention it to an employee. There are predictable patterns that rumors will follow. The most crucial details, such as store closings and subsequent loss of jobs, will be sharpened. These will become the central part of repeated communications of the rumor. These details will become intensified. The plans to downsize or close three stores will grow to 10 stores in repeated retellings. The number of jobs affected will increase from a small number to 50 or more.

Aspects of Jack's thinking that seem peripheral and that might lessen the emotional impact of the rumor will be downplayed, a process known as *leveling*. For example, Jack's plan to wait for people to begin their school shopping will be eliminated from the rumor, much as bumps in hills will be leveled prior to building a road. The resulting rumor will be short, precise, and easy to communicate in everyday language. Rumors will also be combined with other impressions and stories that are circulating within an organization. If workers have observed that Jack seems to be very friendly with a female store manager, then the rumors will include the observation that her job is safe. These additional details are likely to be colorful, intriguing, or to use nontechnical language, "juicy."

The way to combat rumors is to provide substitutes for them in the form of clear and helpful communications (Eisenberg, 2007). Realizing that rumors are unpreventable, Jack should let his employees know about company problems and what is being done to address them. This action has the additional advantage of stimulating suggestions from employees concerning ways to increase sales and customer service.

USING OUR COGNITIVE ABILITIES: THE CASE OF PUBLIC SPEAKING

When consulting with people in organizations, I frequently appeal to how they can think more effectively about problems, stressors, and other workplace difficulties. I often begin conversations with questions about what managers find enjoyable and unenjoyable. When focusing on tasks that they particularly dislike, many managers complain about making oral presentations in the workplace. They are nervous about being poorly prepared. They are anxious about being the center of attention. They feel that executives are judging them against the standards of the most effective public speakers in the organization. They feel that managers at their same level would like to see them fail so that there will be less competition during the next round of promotions. When managers ask, I give them advice about reducing stress and anxiety (Lazarus & Folkman, 1984). First, I suggest that they obtain experience speaking in front of others. If they attend church services regularly, they could volunteer to do readings. If they are active in youth sports, they can voice their concerns at organizational meetings attended by parents and other community volunteers. If they have some free evenings, they can take courses in public speaking offered through university outreach programs.

Managers can also benefit from research studies that have investigated the components of effective public presentations (Allen & Preiss, 1998; Petty & Brinol, 2008; Petty, Wheeler, & Tormala, 2003). In organizations, many presentations deal in some way with planned changes or modifications in the way that people go about their work. For example, an organization might be planning to change its software for the management of inventory. There are often both positive aspects and negative aspects of any proposed change. Positive aspects might be that the new software is easier to use and that it provides clear visual displays of various kinds of inventory. With the software, it will be easy to identify materials that the company needs to purchase. Negative aspects might be the cost of the software, the time needed to train workers in its use, and the resistance from workers who are perfectly happy with the old software.

Speakers often ask, "Should I present just the positive reasons for my recommendations concerning change, or should I present both the plusses and minuses?" When members of the audience are intelligent and well versed in the matter under discussion, the answer is "both positive and negative." With this decision, speakers communicate that they are well prepared and sophisticated enough to know that all recommendations for change come with a downside. Speakers are also giving credit to their audience since experienced executives know that change involves plusses and minuses. As one executive told me, "I always recommend that both sides of an issue be covered. If people say that there are no downsides to their recommendations, sophisticated audience members will not believe them."

Another advantage of covering both sides of an issue is that it takes speakers' attention away from their anxiety and nervousness. If they invest the effort necessary to do a thorough job covering both the advantages and disadvantages of their recommendations, they will experience the self-confidence that comes from being well prepared. If they focus on thoughts such as "I must be sure to highlight both pluses and minuses," then they will not be focusing on thoughts such as "I feel tense and nervous."

When people focus on the content of their presentation and the feelings surrounding the hard work they invested in preparing their talks, they engage in a process called thought distraction (Vassilopoulos, 2008). An old song comes to mind. In *The King and I*, Anna tells her students that when she is anxious, "I whistle a happy tune, so no one will suspect I'm afraid." As well as making a good impression on others, people who engage in distracting activities may also convince themselves that they are comfortable with their tasks.

At times, the distracting activity can involve imagining settings where people are comfortable in public. In high school, I participated in the drama club and acted in plays. Any fear of appearing in public lessened as the cast rehearsed plays again and again and as people memorized their lines. When I first started speaking in public on a regular basis, I imagined myself as an actor in a play. Since I had become comfortable in my role as actor, focusing on this activity reduced my anxiety about giving a speech in public.

Some people are known to be good storytellers at family gatherings. When giving a talk in public, they could imagine themselves telling stories to familiar and appreciative people at a family party. Further, they can think of the audience for their speech as family members whom they have known all their lives. By engaging in this step, they are taking advantage of a fact about public presentations. Most audience members want to like the speaker. They do not want to be bored and they want the speaker to be successful. If speakers imagine that audience members want to be appreciative, this is another technique that can reduce their anxiety.

This presentation on thought processes surrounding public speaking provides a good introduction to the next chapter. Almost everything we do in the workplace involves other people, whether those people are coworkers, superiors, subordinates, or customers. We need to understand others, to work smoothly with them, and to form group ties.

4

Groups in the Workplace

INTRODUCTION

We need other people in our lives. Very few of us would be happy living as hermits in a cave, cut off from the rest of society. Other people provide a wide range of resources (Kurzman, 2009). They offer social support when we are stressed, information about various life opportunities, company when we feel lonely, and additions to our talents when we work with them on complex projects (Hamniton & Hewstone, 2007).

Other people help us satisfy our needs, but we must contribute to the satisfaction of their needs, goals, and desires. If we only interact with people for self-benefit, we will be dismissed as leeches, users, and takers. Addressing the satisfaction of our needs with contributions to the needs of other is a delicate balancing act (Buss, 2008). Some people do it better than others. For people who do it very well, expectations of large salaries and the titles of manager, president, and chief executive officer can become realities (Kinicki & Williams, 2008).

Students in all accredited business schools take a mandatory course in management. No matter what their major (e.g., accounting, finance, information technology), students are expected to take a solid course on basic issues involving management in organizations. Much of the course deals with how best to work with other people. A typical four-part outline (Kinicki & Williams, 2008) is: managers plan for the future with others in the organization, they organize people so that organizational goals are met, they provide leadership, and they evaluate whether or not people's activities are contributing to goal achievement.

On the first day that students meet, professors are fond of introducing the class with a statement such as the following: "Professors who teach this course realize that you might be enrolled only because it is a requirement. We hope that, after the course is completed, you will feel that it has been a good use of your time. What you learn in this course may not be what leads to your first job. Your first set of job offers might be based on technical skills you have learned, such as tax auditing and the ability to design a questionnaire for a marketing survey. But what you learn in this class will be central to your future in any company 10 years from now. Will you be promoted, or will you be at the same level as when you were hired? Will you enter the ranks of management and leadership in your organization, with corresponding higher salaries? Will you be asked to represent your company in community-wide forums and at national and international professional meetings? The answers to these questions will depend on how well you work with other people, and this is a major topic within the required business school management course."

GROUPS AND SURVIVAL

People have a special sensitivity to their interactions with others and to the formation of groups (Van Vugt et al., 2008). In our ancestral past, no one person could survive by himself or herself. A small group of hunters might be successful one day, but not on another. Survival would be increased if each small group developed norms that involved the sharing of resources. One group, if successful on a hunt, would share food with others. As part of this sharing, group members would expect reciprocity if another small band of hunters was successful next week. Cheaters, or those who did not reciprocate, would run the risk of being ostracized. Similar survival value would be attached to other resources such as the availability of edible plants, access to potential mates, and technical skills such as tool making (Buss, 2008). The concept "you do something for me and I'll do something for you" has a long history among human beings.

The essential role that other people play in survival helps explain a question that many readers have had about teenagers. I certainly had the same question as I participated in the raising of three children during their adolescent years. Why is a peer group so important to teenagers? Why are adolescents so sensitive to rejection by their age peers? Why do they want to be accepted by others of the same age, even sometimes defying parents in their quest for peer approval? One answer to the questions stems from our distant ancestral past. Thousands of years ago, what were teenagers likely to be? The answer is "orphans." Given life expectancy in our ancestral past, many people did not live past 30 years of age. This meant that they would be leaving teenage children behind. For these orphaned teenagers, the chances of survival would increase if they banded together and shared resources with each other. If one had an elderly uncle who provided food, this would be shared with others in the peer group. If one learned adult skills such as tool making quicker than others, he or she would pass on the skills. If one knew of a plant that would help with a medical problem, this information could be shared. Individuals who did not become attached to an adolescent peer group would not receive such resources and might not survive. Current adolescent concerns about peer acceptance (which were the same for readers of this book during their teenage years) are a remnant of a mechanism for survival.

THE FORMATION OF GROUPS

One reason that people must come together in organization and form effective groups also deals with survival, in this case the survival of the organization (Greenberg & Baron, 2008). The challenges facing businesses today are so complex that individual employees must be able to combine their talents with those of others and to form groups. Employers are asking the faculty of business schools to prepare students to work in groups. Job applicants will often be asked questions about their group memberships and their contributions to various work teams.

Groups are collections of people who influence one another. Effective groups combine the skills of individual members and encourage the development of innovative contributions that go beyond the abilities of any one person. The influential social scientist George Homans (1950) suggested that groups have four features. Members of groups interact with each other. Further, they listen and respond to each other's messages during their communications. Person A contributes, person B takes that into account and offers suggestions, and person B in turn recognizes A's efforts. This is quite different from people speaking without any reference to the presence of others.

If they are members of groups, people engage in mutually agreed-on activities. In the workplace, these activities involve goals that cannot be achieved by one person and demand collective effort. Examples are bringing a new product to market, organizing a convention, and developing complex software. While activities are often accomplished most effectively through face-to-face meetings, more and more "virtual groups" are working together given today's computer technology. I know of team projects that have been successfully completed through e-mail, and the group members never had a face-to-face meeting.

Group members develop affective ties, also called sentiments. In effective groups, the sentiments are positive and respectful. Problems arise when negative emotions come to the forefront; groups suffering from negativity are likely to become unproductive and dysfunctional. People who work in groups agree to behave according to shared norms that guide their everyday behaviors (Sherif, 1966). Norms exist for various aspects of the workplace: punctuality, informal indicators of who is productive and who is not, and the amount of nonwork-socializing that is expected. Groups often have leaders who are "rate setters." These people model what group members have agreed is a reasonable work load and level of productivity. Some ambitious newcomers to a workplace become "rate busters" if they go beyond the group norm regarding productivity. These people risk becoming socially rejected and will find themselves uninvited to informal group gatherings. Some people can accept this isolation and some cannot. If they are to become group members, these newcomers must become attentive to the agreed-on workplace norms.

Company executives who view employees as individuals who work only for their narrow and independent self-interests are mistaken. Groups exert powerful influences on members, and executives should recognize their importance in the workplace (Borman, 2004). Change efforts should often focus on group norms as well as the goals of individual workers.

HELPFUL INDIVIDUAL TRAITS FOR INTERACTING WITH OTHERS

Some people, perhaps because of genetic gifts and perhaps because of childhood and adolescent experiences that involved extensive interactions with peers and adults, are more skillful than others at encouraging the formation of effective groups. Both intrapersonal and interpersonal skills are necessary. Especially when pronounced quickly, these two terms may sound the same, but there are important distinctions.

The terms refer to different skills that managers should bring to their workplaces. *Interpersonal skills* refer to how well managers get along with people, whether they are able to show respect for the contributions of employees, and whether they are sensitive to the viewpoints of others (Brewer, 2007); Kurzban & Neubeerg, 2005; Thomas & Inkson, 2009). Such skills include listening carefully, not interrupting others and finishing their sentences, and demonstrating genuine concern when employees have problems. Many times, employees will have concerns but will be uncomfortable bringing them to the attention of their bosses. Managers with interpersonal skills will sense when employees have such difficulties and will encourage them to share their viewpoints (Fisher & Ury, 1983). Such managers develop a sensitivity that is much like an antenna that picks up subtle signals concerning employee problems.

Employees want to work for managers who show respect for their past experiences, qualifications, and contributions. When people do not share the same cultural background, there can be difficulties because people may not attach the same value to certain experiences and qualifications. Managers from the mainland sometimes have problems in Hawaii. They may have gone to prestigious private universities and may have worked in New York City and Washington, D.C. If they move to Hawaii and look at the resumes of locals, they will find that many have not lived for long periods of time on the mainland. Further, the job experiences that locals list may be unfamiliar to mainland managers. This unfamiliarity can lead to judgments that locals have not had experiences that are sufficiently challenging or important. Such managers often have a short tenure in Hawaii because they are unable to show respect for others. If they remain in Hawaii, they learn that their mainland experiences are likely to be different but are not necessarily better.

Intrapersonal skills refer to knowledge about the self and the ability to view oneself objectively (George, 2000; Moon, 2003). Managers with intrapersonal skills can ask questions such as, ''How am I coming across to my employees? Am I being overbearing? Am I demonstrating that I have respect for their work? How could I improve as a manager?'' The development of intrapersonal skills requires a great deal of self-insight. Somehow, people find it easy to comment on other people's problems but are blind to their own shortcomings. Some managers develop intrapersonal skills through feedback sessions with trusted mentors. For example, after an especially busy and stressful month, managers might ask senior executives to give them constructive feedback on how they handled themselves under pressure.

If managers want to improve, they can if they are willing to invest time and effort. For example, if they have the intrapersonal knowledge that they often come across as aloof, they can practice behaviors that could challenge this reputation. They might try self-deprecating humor or do volunteer work in community organizations where they will interact with employees as equals (Brislin, 1991).

ENCOURAGING PARTICIPATION

Good managers must direct the talents of others into activities that assist in the accomplishment of organizational goals (Pencavel, 2003; Strauss, 2006). An old image of managers, perhaps more myth than reality, is that they could do any job in the organization. If an

employee was sick, for instance, the manager could pitch in and perform the duties of the absent worker. This image is no longer useful.
Today's organizations are so complex that no one person can possibly
have the skills needed for multiple jobs. In a large department store,
for instance, different people must have detailed knowledge about
sales, various product lines, information technology, accounting, personnel policies, finance, and marketing to previously untapped demographic groups. These multiple needs of the modern organization
require managers who can supervise employees who have more
knowledge and skills about specific aspects of the organization.

If employees have relevant knowledge of use to the organization,
today's managers should be able to encourage workers to share their
insights and to participate in company decision making. There are
many benefits when employees participate. They share their knowledge
both with managers and with coworkers. Many times, workers discover effective work techniques through their everyday trial and error,
and these insights should be shared with others. Participation in company decision making also encourages a feeling that employees share
company goals and the paths to achieving these goals. If employees
buy into a company vision through their active participation, they are
likely to work hard toward achieving the vision.

Companies sometimes have difficulties moving from a centralized
and authoritarian decision-making type to one that is more participative (Cummins, 2005). If workers are not accustomed to speaking up
and sharing their ideas, time is needed to make them more comfortable
with these tasks. Executives cannot enter a room, announce the change
to participative decision making, and then expect workers to suggest
lots of new ideas. Employees must learn to be comfortable speaking up
in front of others. In my experience, outside consultants are often
brought in to introduce various public-speaking and team-building
skills. If a company's decision making has been highly centralized, the
change to a more open, democratic, and participative style can take a
year or longer.

Employees must also trust that management will use the products of
their participation in a just and ethical manner (Greenberg, 1997).
Often, workers feel that if they speak up with suggestions, thin-skinned
managers will take these as criticisms of the status quo. Further,
employees feel that managers may retaliate if they do not approve of
the suggestions. If a company has a history of difficult management-
labor relations, trust can take a long time to develop. Employees may
make a few "trial suggestions" to see how management reacts (Brislin,
1991). If leaders demonstrate that they are using the suggestions and
that they are sincere about worker participation, employees will note
this and make more contributions to decision making in the future.

OVERCOMING DIFFICULTIES BROUGHT ON BY GROUPS

The major advantage of working effectively in groups is that the talents of any one person can be complemented by the abilities and contributions of others (Halevy & Sagiv, 2008). Projects that could not be undertaken or completed by one person become possible when the efforts of several people can be integrated. Further, the positive feelings generated by thoughts such as "this group is important to me" and "we are all in this together" can direct people toward actions beneficial to an organization.

Difficulties can arise, however, when people form groups. Three such difficulties are that (1) people will conform to group decisions even if one or more individuals feel that the decision is wrong; (2) as a result, they may engage in groupthink (Janis, 1982) that leads to overconfidence in initial preferences and too little effort invested in searches for various possible recommendations for eventual decision making. As part of their decision making, (3) people often engage in riskier alternatives as group members than they would as individual actors. This can lead to positive outcomes, such as, encouragement to accept the risk inherent in entrepreneurial ventures, but it can also lead to severe problems, such as teenage drinking and driving.

Conformity. People often go along with the wishes of a group, even if they think the group is wrong, because they do not want to stand out as dissenters, killjoys, wet blankets, or whiners. Imagine this experience (from Asch, 1956). People volunteer for a research study on the perception of learning materials. They are told that they will be examining various ways of presenting information and that they will give their opinions on which ways are clear and which are not. These materials will include visual presentations on chalkboards, overhead transparencies, and PowerPoint slides. The importance of the study is emphasized. Researchers explain that in this fast-moving world, people must learn about new technologies very quickly or else their job skills will become outdated. Finding effective ways of presenting information in workplace training sessions is essential.

The people who volunteer for the study enter a room. There are eight participants, and they sit in a single row toward the front of a classroom. On a chalkboard they see one line on the left of the board and eight lines on the right. The researcher says, "To begin the study, I need to know how big the material presented on the chalkboard needs to be so that everyone can see it clearly. Could you tell me which of the lines on the right hand side of the chalkboard is the same size as the single line on the left?" People then give their answers. There is one person whose answers are of interest to the researchers. This is the seventh person in the row. Before he answers, six people give their answer concerning the length of the lines. From the seventh person's point of view, the first six are wrong. They are clearly making a mistake when they give their report concerning the equal size of lines on the left- and right-hand sides of the chalkboard. It is now time for the seventh person to give his response. What does he do? Does he report what he thinks is the correct answer, or does he go along with the incorrect answer given by the first six respondents?

As first reported by Solomon Asch (1956), many people set aside their own correct response and report the incorrect answer given by the first six respondents. This study, which has been widely replicated, shows the power of groups on the behavior of individuals. Groups set norms, or shared standards of acceptable behavior. If people go against group norms and become nonconformists, there can be sanctions. Nonconformists are often shunned by others (Homans, 1950). They find themselves uninvited to social gatherings. They can be treated by others as odd or weird. In the workplace, nonconformists find that they are ignorant of information passed along through grapevines since nobody talks to them regularly (Monsour-Cole & Scott, 1998; Van Hoye & Lievens, 2009).

People work hard at avoiding the status of social pariahs by attending to the standards that are established by their groups. They work hard to fit in as best they can so that they do not become social deviants and do not become the targets of gossip (Homans, 1950). The need to "fit in" and to avoid social ostracism is very strong (Sherif, 1966). Even though the seventh person in the perception study was not previously acquainted with any of the first six respondents, he may have gone along with the group so that he would not be seen as odd, stupid, or deviant. Even when people go against the group and give the correct answer, they are clearly upset that they are disagreeing with six other people. While giving their correct answer they fidget, look at the others to see their reactions, and show discomfort in their facial expressions.

This research shows the power of group norms (Goldstone, Roberts, & Gureckis, 2008). In the workplace, employees observe the behavior of coworkers and are attentive to norms concerning productivity, workloads, and willingness to take on extra assignments. Managers who want to see changes such as increased productivity or greater use of technology are wise to examine people's work affiliations. Many times, managers need to change group norms if they want to introduce workplace changes.

Groupthink. In this classic study by Asch (1956), people who participated in the experiment were not acquainted with others who were working on the same task. The mere presence of others who might frown and ridicule any one person was enough to encourage conformity among many participants. Problems can increase when people know each other well.

When people work with each other for long periods of time, they often form close ties and strong emotional bonds. When they come together to make decisions, they may consider various alternatives. Often, however, there are pressures to go along with what is clearly a favored position. This recommendation for action may be preferred by the highest-ranking executive, a colleague who has recently done favors for people, or an especially popular individual. When people do not consider various alternatives and go along with the group so as to maintain workplace harmony, they are guilty of *groupthink*.

This term, coined by Irving Janis (1982), refers to uncritical thinking that is meant to maintain closeness within the group. Consider a meeting where managers, who have worked with each other for 10 or more years, are considering introducing a new product line. Several of the managers have put in extensive time and energy into work on this issue, and they recommend steps to begin manufacturing, quality control, and marketing. But two of the group members have reservations. One feels that the new product line cannot be protected by patents. Consequently, competitors can quickly introduce "knockoffs," and this will confuse the company's longtime customers. Another manager feels that insufficient attention has been given to employee safety concerns given the new manufacturing processes that will be introduced. Will the two doubters speak up? The pressures they face are a major part of groupthink analysis.

Group members place pressures on those who disagree. At times, there will be appeals to loyalty. There will be reminders of good group decisions made in the past. There can be reminders of outside pressures, such as investors' disappointment with performance of the company's stock in recent months. Another reason people do not speak up is that they feel "the train has left the station." So many people support the decision that group members feel enthusiastic about moving ahead in a positive direction. Individuals who bring up objections may be perceived as malcontents, killjoys, and troublemakers.

Good executives, recognizing the possibility of groupthink, take steps to overcome it (Janis, 1982). I have been at meetings where the leader has said, "I don't hear any objections to this proposal. This is bad, because it may mean that we are not considering all alternatives and are frittering away opportunities to improve the proposal." Other executives appoint a manager who takes the role of the devil's advocate (Grout & Fisher, 2007). To fulfill the role, the manager must bring in reasons why the proposal is not a good idea. If the person does a half-hearted job and does little more than support the proposal through weak counterarguments, this will be reflected in the manager's performance evaluation. The goal of this exercise is to make sure that all positive and negative aspects of various proposals have been thoroughly examined. Many times, thoughtful objections are integrated into revisions of the proposal, and the improvements increase the chances of eventual company success.

Good managers can deal with some of the negative outcomes of conformity and groupthink by encouraging employees willing to make suggestions at odds with group preferences. The managers need to know, however, that nonconformists face great pressures. People do not enjoy the reputation of being group deviants. There are social sanctions that are directed at nonconformists. They find themselves uninvited to social gatherings. At work, others go off to lunch in a group and leave the nonconformist behind. Even if their ideas are good, group deviants find that no one is willing to speak out to support their proposals. In extreme circumstances, sanctions are directed at the nonconformists' children. As discussed earlier in this chapter, all readers will remember how important it was to be accepted by others during their junior high and high school years. Imagine the unhappiness of students if they find no one to eat lunch with in the school cafeteria. If this dreaded occurrence is due to the outspokenness of their parents, then family strife is certain. Many parents have given in at this point. "I can take being treated like a pariah because of my opinions, but I cannot stand to see my children being the targets of social rejection."

So what are the possible decisions facing people who have opinions that differ from group norms? Should they just go along with the group, or should they stick to their opinions? While there is no piece of advice that will be helpful to everyone, here is a suggestion that may sometimes be of use: People can consider making contributions to the group that are independent of the disagreements that led to the original conformity pressures (Hollander, 1992). Let's use the example of disagreements concerning how a volunteer organization is to use its funds. Most members want to spend excess funds on a college scholarship. One person, Angie Chen, speaks in favor of donating the money to a private elementary school that assists disabled students. Angie will get a better hearing if she has made previous contributions to the group. She may have organized fund-raisers, headed recruiting drives for new members, and volunteered for cleanup duty as part of the group's yearly banquet.

To use a phrase coined by the Edwin Hollander (1992), a person who contributes to a group builds up "idiosyncrasy credit." That is, contributors build up good will through their actions. If a time comes when they feel that they must be a nonconformist and must argue against a group consensus, then they are given some slack. Their non-conformity is seen as an idiosyncratic or odd act which does not merit rejection since they have made so many group contributions. Efforts on behalf of the group have another advantage. Members might say, "Angie has done a lot for the group and clearly values her membership. She disagrees with us on this issue, but we should respect her and listen to her ideas."

Risk Taking. When people interact in groups, their initial attitudes and preferences are often intensified (Kogan & Wallach, 1964). For example, individuals might examine the possibility of purchasing a franchise that is part of a successful restaurant chain. After extensive research, they decide that the restaurant has a reasonable chance of success, but still have doubts about investing their time and money. Then, these individuals discuss the franchising possibility with other knowledgeable people. The potential buyer and the others meet as a group. If the individuals were leaning toward purchasing the franchise, they will be more likely to follow through on their intentions after the group discussion.

Researchers who have investigated this type of communication and decision making first called it *the risky shift phenomenon* (Kogan & Wallach, 1964). Individuals are more likely to make risky decisions after interacting with others and engaging in a group discussion. One reason for the risky shift is that more information becomes available during the group discussion. One group member may tell the investor, "Even if the restaurant is not successful, you will learn a great deal about starting your own business." Another might say, "The restaurant chain already has ads on TV and people in this community have seen them." A second reason is that group members remind the potential investor about values that are commonly held by members of the larger society. Risk taking and entrepreneurship are highly valued in the United States, and the presence of others reminds the decision-makers that risks can lead to rewards.

After the initial studies carried out in the United States, researchers investigated decision making in other countries. In some traditional African cultures, there is value placed on tradition and to the conservative norms that have led to success and survival in the past. In these cultures, children are taught to admire people with traditional knowledge. For example, there may be elders who know of edible plants that are not tasty and that are not part of people's everyday diets. However, knowledge of these plants is very useful when other food is unavailable and people face starvation. In these traditional cultures, individuals often make more conservative decisions after discussions with group members.

Researchers then made adjustments to the language used to summarize their findings (Hong, 1978). They changed the term *risky shift* to *value shift*. If a culture values risk, this will be the direction in which group decisions move. If a culture values conservatism and tradition, this will be the direction that groups take.

The change to value shift suggested that researchers should look at different areas of decision making within a country. On issues of personal safety, for example, Americans are likely to avoid risks. Few people would accept the removal of today's elaborate screening procedures in airports. They will not be influenced because statisticians argue that the risk of terrorism is low on any one specific flight. When a danger is clear in people's minds, the traditional wisdom captured by the term *safety first* guides decision making.

Whenever issues of risk and decision making arise, discussions often move toward their relation to legalized gambling (Cummins, Nadorff, & Kelly, 2009; Gupta, Derevensky, & Ellenbogen, 2006). Many people from all parts of North America travel to Las Vegas and Reno and risk money in the hopes of winning more. Others, who themselves do not gamble, are fascinated by the amount of travel to Nevada and liken it to pilgrimages. What's the difference between the two groups?

I should mention that my experiences with casino gambling are very limited. On a trip to Australia, I played the one-cent slots in a casino along the Gold Cost. I wagered about ten cents in all, and can't remember if I came away a winner or not.

People who travel regularly to Vegas are willing to take risks. They often have friends who make the same trip. So when one person is contemplating a trip, there will almost surely be relatives and friends who say, "Great idea! Maybe this is the time you'll win big!" Consequently, the person has his or her initial tendency reinforced and is more likely to take the trip than to visit the Liberace Museum or the Hoover Dam. On the other hand, people who do not gamble regularly often associate with people who have similar outlooks.

At the University of Hawaii, for instance, I know very few people who gamble regularly. Most faculty members I know are well versed in statistics. If I told them that I was considering a trip to Vegas but thought that San Francisco might be more interesting, they would reinforce this inclination. They would say, "You're right to lean toward Frisco. Keep in mind that most people who gamble in Vegas lose money. They did not build the Venetian and the Luxor by making sure that people left Vegas with more money than they came with!"

Some people who are willing to take risks find outlets for their motives other than gambling. For example, people may attach their risk-taking propensities to an entrepreneurial venture in the business world. If they are good writers, they may turn down a salaried job and instead hope for royalties from magazine articles or novels. Or, they may find an outlet in certain sports such as parachute jumping, surfing 15-foot waves, or motorcycle racing. As with the examples of gamblers and people who have never seen the inside of a casino, these risk takers are likely to have friends who share the same interests and who will urge the individuals to move ahead with their plans.

INGROUPS AND OUTGROUPS

Whenever people who share the same interests (for example, gambling) come together, they may form a group that excludes those who do not share their interests. This can lead to a dysfunctional workplace where employees do not know whether they are in the groups most favored by management.

Other reasons for forming groups beyond shared interests include ethnicity, shared physical characteristics, and the holding of similar opinions (Allport, 1954; Brewer, 2007). People in one's ingroup share perceived similarities. People have positive feelings about members of their ingroups and enjoy interacting with them. Individuals in one's outgroup are different in some way. They look different, have a language or accent that can't be understood, think differently, or behave in ways considered unacceptable to the person making judgments about group membership (Brislin, 2008).

The formation of ingroups and outgroups is universal and is a basic fact that marks human beings, similar to the needs for food, water, and sleep (Buss, 2008). Many people make decisions about their behavior based on their ingroups and outgroups. For example, we might consider all candidates running for elective office and vote for those who will best represent all the people in our state. But we don't. Instead, we divide candidates into ingroups and outgroups. In some states such as Hawaii, California, and Florida, the ethnic vote (my group and other groups) is a factor that politicians must consider if they are to be elected. When executives favor candidates from certain ethnic groups for jobs in their organizations, they are behaving according to ingroup and outgroup distinctions. Such choices are sometimes unconscious. The executives simply prefer candidates who share similarities and who seem familiar.

The danger of ingroup and outgroup formation is that others considered different are sometimes put at a disadvantage in their quest for society's benefits (Brewer, 2007; Triandis, 2009). Denying resources to outgroup members is common when people express prejudiced attitudes toward others who are different. Various forms of prejudice include racism, tokenism, interference with a culture's values, and judging others based on one's real likes and dislikes (Brislin, 2000). Other ingroup and outgroup distinctions are based on what is familiar and unfamiliar to people. These distinctions are especially prominent when people move from one city to another and must learn new behaviors that will allow them to satisfy everyday needs. People moving from the mainland United States to Hawaii, for example, face the need to engage in many unfamiliar behaviors. Examples are attending baby luaus, learning new terms such as *pau* (finished or completed), *hapa* (half), and *niele* (nosy, overly intrusive with one's curiosity), and making sure that others do not lose face during interpersonal interactions.

The inclusion of the familiar and unfamiliar in discussions of intergroup relations may seem out of place. Prejudices based on racist beliefs seem far removed from ingroup-outgroup misunderstandings based on unfamiliar behaviors. I include them in the same discussion because the outcomes are similar. People from different groups do not interact frequently or smoothly. They are not benefiting from the stimulation provided when diverse people interact, share their varied perspectives, and arrive at decisions that are better because people have integrated complex viewpoints (Thomas, Ravlin, & Wallace, 1996).

Ingroup and outgroup misunderstandings based on unfamiliar behaviors are relatively easy to address (Brislin & Yoshida, 1994). In a diverse workplace, for example, executives can ask the question, "What are differences that, over the years, have caused misunderstandings among people here in the workplace?" In a large organization, human resource specialists can be brought in to add to the list of differences. Then, these differences can be explained to everyone as part of formal training programs, mentoring activities in the workplace, and during informal conversations among people (Singelis, 1998).

AVOIDING REACTANCE

Much of this chapter is aimed at helping managers deal with the additional skills necessary to deal with groups. Managers may be skillful when working with individual employees but less effective when those employees form groups and thus add dynamics such as norm formation to the workplace. Another dynamic that managers should know is that employees resent unreasonable efforts that threaten their freedom of action (Brehm, 1966). We can start a discussion of this topic with a critical incident.

People Resent Attempts to Interfere with Their Preferred Behaviors

At the company where Paul Cummings worked, the chief executive officer formed a panel to consider applications for promotions. Paul served on this panel along with six other managers. Paul had a reputation in the company for holding strong opinions and for being quick to share them with others. At the actual selection meeting, committee members reviewed the applications of three candidates for a newly created managerial position that dealt with Web-based marketing. Paul argued strongly for his preferred candidate. He used a loud and forceful tone of voice, was very intense with his body language, and he rose from his seat several times to write down the reasons for his preference on a chalkboard.

Paul took so much time defending his candidate that other selection committee members had few opportunities to speak. When one other member used the little time she had to discuss another candidate, Paul seemed disinterested and looked at his watch several times. At the end of the meeting, the committee members wrote down their preferences on secret ballots and placed them in a box. Later, when the results of the vote were announced, Paul was displeased to learn that his preferred candidate received only two votes.

Paul has encountered an example of reactance (Brehm, 1966). When people have freedoms taken away from them, they react in a negative manner. The people then seek out attempts to reassert their freedoms and to behave in ways of their own choosing. Parents are familiar with this phenomenon. They present their preferences to their teenage children: obey curfews, don't drink alcohol, don't drive above the speed limit, make sure your homework is done before talking to friends on cell phones. But teenagers often react in a negative manner. They feel that some of their cherished freedoms are being taken away by their unreasonable parents. So they make attempts to reassert their freedoms through behaviors that they freely choose. They make choices to be careless about curfews, alcohol use, freeway driving, and homework. Reactance can be especially problematic with adolescents whose ability to think about the consequences of behaviors is not fully developed (Butters, 2005).

In the case of the selection committee considering candidates for promotion, Paul is interfering with people's freedoms. These freedoms include speaking up in favor of one's preferred candidate, engaging in mature and professional discussion of issues, and listening to the opinions of all selection committee members. Paul took up so much time during the meeting that he did not give others opportunities to speak and to communicate with one another. The others then made attempts to reassert themselves. When members of the selection committee filled out their secret ballots, they voted for the candidates they felt were the best qualified, and their preferences were different from Paul's.

In democratic elections, reactance is common when there is bombastic rhetoric concerning a referendum or political candidate. People can be quiet and passive when listening to the rhetoric. But their silence should not be taken as agreement with the positions being argued or the candidates being touted. People can very quietly go to the privacy of voting booths and voice opinions opposite to those that have been voiced by loud and vociferous activists. At times, they will assert their freedom by making a point of voting against the positions and candidates favored by the most strident and most boisterous activists (Sherif, Sherif, & Nebergall, 1965).

Good managers are aware of a fact not possessed by poor managers: Everyone wants respect (Grant & Mayer, 2009; Grout & Fisher, 2007). Problems of not receiving enough respect became a major part of Rodney Dangerfield's comedy routines. As part of their reaction to disrespect and inattention from others, people often become even more convinced of their original positions. One reason is that people react negatively toward the tactics of their proponents. They say, "If these other people have nothing to offer but the ability to interrupt and to be condescending, then we are certainly not going to move toward their position." If the opponents made some good points, as they did in the example of the discussion about job candidates, these would be overlooked given negative feelings concerning the opponents' presentation style. People are attentive to both what others say and how they say it, and the manner in which the others state their positions often takes precedence.

Reactance can be seen when athletic teams prepare for games. One team says that their opponents are soft and are a bunch of chokers. The team that is the target of these jibes becomes even more convinced that they will win the game and they put more energy into preparations. Often, in postgame interviews, members of the winning team say that they were fired up as a result of their opponents' trash talk. For this reason, coaches tell their players to be careful what they say about opponents prior to game time.

Reactance can be minimized if people listen carefully and respectfully to the arguments of those who disagree with them. People can be firm when presenting their opinions to others who are likely to disagree, but they should do so in a calm, reasoned manner (Brislin, 1991). After listening respectfully to the others, people can acknowledge any good points that are raised. When people listen carefully, they often find points of agreement around which compromises can be based. In the discussions about marketing, for instance, the opponents may bring up issues concerning appropriate media outlets. The proponent may recognize the legitimacy of the concerns and make modifications in their original proposal. All people at the meeting will then feel that they are making contributions and are part of efforts to improve the company. But this exchange of information and concerns cannot take place if people are more interested in shouting and silencing opponents than in forming coalitions in which all concerned individuals can offer mutual support (Lewicki, Saunders, & Barry, 2006).

BENEFITS OF WORKING WELL WITH GROUPS

People become much more effective in their workplaces when they learn to work well with others and to integrate themselves into groups (Homans, 1950; Feeney, 2006; Thomas et al., 1996). I taught in a psychology department in the early 1970s. One of my undergraduate students, although very intelligent, was not concerned about what others thought of her. She criticized others very freely, often in colorful language, had little good to say about her surroundings, and seemed to take up controversial causes just for the sake of rebelliousness. Just a few years ago, I spotted her name on a Web site for a university where she worked and where I once went to school. She has an uncommon name, so I used the Google search engine, found an e-mail address, and contacted her to ask if she was the same person who took my course. She was. She is now a university vice president. When I was in the city where she lives, we had lunch. I asked her, "What advice do you think I should give my current students based on your career success?" Her response was, "Work well with other people and gain their respect." Remembering her past behaviors, I asked, "When did you learn this?" Her answer was, "Late!" I followed up: "About what age were you?" Her answer, "Late!" She said this word with a firm tone of voice, and while remaining socially skillful and appropriately gentle, she still communicated the message that she would like to change the topic. My guess is that she was well into her thirties before she figured out the importance of good relations with others and the importance of working well in groups.

I have lived in Hawaii for over 35 years, and good relationships are central to doing good business in this state. I feel that observations about Hawaii are similar to any relatively small community where people knew each other 10 years ago and expect to interact with the same individuals 10 years from now.

Good Business Relationships. When asked about formulating plans for a successful business, experienced executives often emphasize location. Further, they use the rhetorical device of repeating this word three times to communicate its importance. When asked the same question in Hawaii, executives do not downplay location and they constantly remind young businesspeople of its central role in good planning. But in addition, they emphasize that successful businesses in Hawaii are based on good relationships (Choo, 2004), and they use the same rhetorical technique by repeating the word.

One reason relationships in Hawaii are so important is that locals have interacted with many businesspeople from the Mainland and from Asia. Some become permanent residents and make important contributors to the quality of life in their communities. Others come to Hawaii, spend time here, move elsewhere, and then stay in contact with locals and continue to do business with them. But other people come to Hawaii, become involved in the business world, and then move away with no further contact with locals. Locals sometimes use the term *seagulls* when referring to these people. Seagulls fly in, leave their droppings, and then fly away. And who has to clean up the droppings? The answer is the locals who had dealings with these people skillful in the performance of disappearing acts.

A vice president of a large financial services firm came to my office and discussed a major problem he was facing. He had lived in Hawaii for five years. His organization had designed a one-stop plan that would allow small businesses to have all their financial needs met. His organization would provide multiple services such as traditional banking, checking, investments, tax preparation, loans, and so forth. But he was having trouble getting local businesspeople to give his organization serious consideration. I replied by saying that many businesspeople have long-term relationships with existing financial service institutions such as savings and loan organizations and small tax preparation companies. These relationships sometimes go back two and three generations, with one person's grandfather working with a colleague's great uncle. Locals often have very specific memories of people with whom they have been doing business for years, such as individuals who offered loans during difficult times when no one else would offer any sort of help.

In addition, I introduced the concept of seagulls. Businesspeople in Hawaii are used to seeing people come and go, and they are wary of newcomers with great-sounding deals. Even if locals agree to do business with the financial services firm, what are the guarantees that they will be working with the same people five years from now? In addition, locals are concerned that they will be seen as disloyal to longtime residents of Hawaii with whom they have done business for many years. Other ties, such as having been classmates in high school, and becoming part of extended families (the commonly used Hawaiian word is *ohanas*) through marriages, also play a big role.

Further discussion centered on the institution's image in Hawaii and perceptions of its employees. Are company managers and executives here for the long term, or will they be leaving just at the point when locals feel comfortable with them (Choo, 2004)? Are company employees becoming involved in volunteer community activities? Are executives from the mainland clearly mentoring young local businesspeople whose families have lived in Hawaii for generations? Are they sensitive to local norms, such as "don't talk stink" and not saying how much better things are on the mainland? Positive answers to these questions are likely to lead to business relationships that will benefit all parties.

Becoming Informed Through Good Relationships. Often, people who are well informed are kept up-to-date because of their positive social relationships (Feeney, 2006).

Personal Relations Can Assist in Cutting through Red Tape

"I can never get any of my paperwork through the administrative office," Steve Lau complained to his friends as he was eating lunch in the company cafeteria. He continued, "No matter what the issue is, travel reimbursements, purchases of equipment, or requests to hire temporary help, there are always delays and memos about rules and regulations that I am not following. I don't want to cheat anyone, I just want my paperwork to move in a timely manner." Steve then addressed one of the others at the lunch table, Charlie Von Epps. "You never complain about paperwork, Charlie! And you always seem to have new equipment and temporary help when we are especially busy." At the end of the lunch hour, Charlie reminded the others that Sylvia Poole in the administrative office was having a birthday next week. Steve did not seem interested in Charlie's news.

Companies can have admittedly detailed and cumbersome administrative procedures, especially for matters requiring monetary expenditures. Legal requirements demanding careful accounting combined with long-standing rules associated with specific companies result in red tape that can frustrate the most patient employees. There are ways, however, of minimizing the burden. One way is for employees such as Steve and Charlie to develop friendly and respectful relationships with people in the administrative office. Charlie seems to have done this, as shown by his statement that Sylvia is having a birthday. Charlie probably has developed a positive relationship with Sylvia, and he remembers events such as birthdays and anniversaries. He may also know of Sylvia's hobbies and can let her know when he reads something in the newspaper that is related to her interests.

Given a positive relationship (Feeney, 2006; Thomas & Inkson, 2009), Charlie is likely to receive help from Sylvia on administrative matters. For example, Sylvia might need more information about a purchase that Charlie wants to make. She could delay her approval until Charlie makes an inquiry, or she could call Charlie and tell him what she needs. Given that she has a positive relationship and knows that she will not be barked at, she is more likely to take this extra step than she is with someone who might give her a sharp retort. Sylvia might also share information about new policies in the organization. People in a company's administrative office often are among the first to hear about developments that have costs associated with them. For example, Sylvia might hear that executives have earmarked money for computer upgrades, and, because of their discussions, knows that Charlie wants a new monitor and some program management software. She might call Charlie to advise him to put his request in as soon as possible.

Another way of cutting through red tape is to have respect for the work of administrative officers (Dierdorf, Rubin, & Morgeson, 2009; Yukl, 2010). It is easy to disparage them with terms such as *bean counters* and *paper pushers*. However, company employees should keep in mind that administrative officers have a tough job. Few people thank them when paperwork for items such as travel reimbursements moves quickly. If they make a mistake on monetary reimbursements, on the other hand, then they have to explain their actions to their supervisors. If administrative officers approve reimbursements with insufficient documentation, then they come under suspicion and their actions will be remembered when they are up for merit raises or promotions. Employees such as Steve and Charlie are well advised to know exactly what administrative officers need and they should provide it in a timely manner. Everyone comes out a winner. Administrative officers can do their jobs, people putting in requests see the paperwork move quickly, and positive relationships in the workplace are nurtured.

5

Challenges to Effective Communication with Others

In today's workplace, there is a prediction that can be made with certainty. People will face challenges when attempting to communicate with others, and they will face challenges when trying to interpret the communications of others (Denhardt, Denhardt, & Aristigueta, 2009). Reasons for potential difficulties include the many reasons that people differ from each other. In the workplace, individuals will interact with others who are different on a variety of dimensions: age, gender, cultural background, personality, interests, intelligence, education, job experience, and a host of other factors (Brislin, 2008). But despite these differences (and sometimes with the ability to benefit from the differences, see Chapter 12), people must find ways to express their opinions, ideas, preferences, and suggestions to others in the workplace. Frustration and stress (Barna, 2009) are guaranteed if people are not able to satisfy their communication goals.

Communication is so important that there are two chapters devoted to the topic in this book. In this chapter, the emphasis will be on potential sources of communication difficulties, including biases in communication (Lilienfeld, Ammirati, & Landfield, 2009), issues where heightened care is needed such as humor (Schnurr, 2009), male-female interactions (Buss, 2008), and the importance of understanding the nature of situational pressures on interpersonal interactions (Zimbardo, 2007). In the following chapters, there will be an emphasis on ways of increasing the probability of effective communication with others given that potential difficulties have been identified. The common thread linking the two chapters is that they deal with the recognition of potential communication difficulties and suggestions concerning how these difficulties can be overcome.

BIASES IN COMMUNICATION

Extensive research has identified numerous potential biases when people communicate with others. Consider this simple diagram of the communication process (see Figure 5.1).

There are many potential stumbling blocks in the process during which a person formulates a message and the end point when a recipient interprets the message. People have biases during the message-formulating step, for instance, when they want to protect their positive self-image or they want to curry favor with powerful people (Chapter 7). There are many types of noise. These include physical noises stemming from heavy traffic or an overly active air conditioner, but they can also include uncertainties stemming from an unfamiliarity with communication norms associated with different age groups, ethnicities, and personalities. The recipient also has goals, such as a preference to maintain a certain image and a certain organized view of the world. Recipients often use their goals as a filter and interpret messages to be consistent with these goals (Beyer, Chattopadhyay, George, Glick, & Pugliese, 1997; Rosenthal & Jacobson, 1968). This is an issue in the following incident.

People Hear What They Want to Hear

The policy research think tank where Kevin Wong worked had experienced budget problems over the last three years. Government cuts and a lackluster economy made contracts hard to obtain. The organization's largest number of contracts dealt with national defense issues. A number of employees, including Kevin, felt that the organization would prosper if executives would make key changes. These employees wanted administrative support that would allow competition for

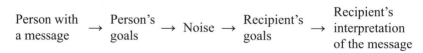

Figure 5.1 The Communication Process

their goal of new contracts in health care research. A new president was recently hired and in her first few weeks made statements such as, "We cannot be wedded so strongly to the past that we miss opportunities for growth." The employees interested in health care were optimistic about change for several months. However, they gradually became disillusioned when the organization continued its emphasis on defense contracts.

Kevin and his like-minded colleagues are victims of the error known as "pulling vague information into a strong category." A more commonly heard phrase is that they heard what they wanted to hear when the new president made statements about "opportunities for growth." People have firmly held opinions, also called strong categories, about different issues (Sherif et al., 1965). Examples are Democratic and Republican affiliations, abortion rights, gun ownership, and increased salaries for public school teachers. Kevin and his colleagues have a strong category concerning expansion into health care research. When influential people make vague statements, listeners pull those statements into their categories. The president talked about the past and how the organization should not be overly attached to it. Kevin pulled this statement into his strongly-held views and felt that the president would approve his recommended move into health research.

The president may have had no such intention in mind. She may have been referring to different types of defense contracts. Perhaps the organization had long been involved in research on how to encourage military personnel to reenlist. She may have in mind moves into other types of defense research, such as training programs for personnel on peacekeeping missions.

Politicians become very skilled at making statements that will attract as many voters as possible (Brislin, 1991). For example, voters have strong opinions pro and con about government-funded health care. If politicians say, "We must do everything possible to provide the best health care for our senior citizens," different people can pull this vague statement toward their position. People in favor of national health insurance will hear support, as will people who want tax breaks for private-sector health care efforts. People can become disappointed and disillusioned if they read too much into the vague statements of executives and politicians. To avoid falling into the trap of hearing what they want to hear, people can ask probing questions and can encourage speakers to be more specific and precise about their proposed policies.

Two Specific Biases: Ego Defensiveness and Naive Realism. When people communicate with others, they want to project a self-image of competence and also want to formulate their messages so that they are persuasive to recipients (De Dreu, 2005). This can lead to two biases that are common during negotiations with others.

Communication Biases Can Derail Negotiations

Having set a goal that labor costs must be reduced, the company for which Lester Martin served as a vice president considered importing goods from China rather than manufacturing them in the United States. Lester's company manufactured and marketed specialized protective clothing products for industries such as home pest extermination, asbestos removal, and laboratory work for technicians who handled potentially dangerous microorganisms. Traveling to Shanghai, Lester met with executives of various Chinese organizations in the hopes of obtaining an agreement for a joint venture. He felt that he had a good business plan that would be attractive to his Chinese counterparts. He pointed out the number of jobs that would be created in Shanghai and the high quality of the housing development he proposed for Chinese workers. Lester was disappointed that the Chinese executives did not share his vision.

The University of Amsterdam's Carsten De Dreu (2005) has identified biases in people's thinking that are especially troublesome during negotiations. Lester may have succumbed to both. One bias is called ego defensiveness. People want to maintain a positive self-view of themselves. They want to view themselves as reasonable individuals who think carefully about problems and who make good decisions. In Lester's case, this positive self-evaluation would include the ability to develop a good business plan that would bring benefits both to his company and to any Chinese company that enters into a joint venture. Given that Lester has had success in his own country, rising to the level of a company vice president, he will be especially anxious to protect his positive self-image.

One way to protect this image is to view others who seem uninterested in his proposal as unreasonable, overly competitive, and incompetent to make good decisions. If Lester feels this way, he is likely to communicate his negative feelings in the course of negotiations with his Chinese counterparts. Since the counterparts also have healthy egos and positive self-evaluations, they may reciprocate the negative feelings. After several rounds of such communications between Lester and his counterparts, the negotiations are likely to spiral into intense negativity. Eventually, they may break down before any agreements are reached.

Another bias in communication is called naïve realism. Negotiations about complex matters are always difficult and stressful. One way that people attempt to cut through the complexity is to simplify the issues under discussion. They can do this by developing a view of reality that is based on the assumption that everyone thinks like they do. Further, they feel that if others don't share their views, then these others are ignorant and unmotivated to contribute to positive changes. Of course, this is naïve: Different people think in a wide variety of ways and have diverse opinions. In Lester's case, he is assuming that his views of what his company can offer China are exactly what the Chinese counterparts want. Lester points to the number of jobs that will be created and the quality of his proposed housing development. The Chinese may be interested in other aspects of a possible joint venture. They may be interested in the amount of job security workers will have and the site of a manufacturing plant. The Chinese may be interested in a plant that will be built in a rural area if they feel that Shanghai is overcrowded and that too many people have moved to the city from small villages.

Steps can be taken to minimize the negative effects of ego defensiveness and naïve realism. De Dreu (2005) suggests that negotiators give attention to four factors. The first is the relative amount of power possessed by the different parties in the negotiation. The second is increasing the accountability of the negotiation process. The third is developing a cooperative rather than competitive orientation during the negotiations. The fourth factor is using time so that the negotiation process starts and continues more productively.

These steps work well when negotiators desire an agreement that meets the interest of all parties involved. The goal of negotiations is not to grind opponents into the dirt or to treat them "as flies to wanton boys" (*King Lear*). The problem with such negotiations is that there will be a party that will label itself the winner, but the loser will not put time and energy into following though on agreements that the winner imposed. Instead, the members of the party not treated well will drag their feet, will challenge the agreements, and in general will work to undermine the efforts of the so-called winner.

If all four factors are given attention during negotiations, people move from being pro-self to pro-social thinkers. That is, they integrate their own interests with those of their counterparts. Further, they engage in careful thinking that has the goal of developing proposals that allow everyone to make progress toward goal achievement. If there is a power balance, one party cannot simply force the other to comply. If people try this, the other party has power of its own and can engage in activities such as resistance, calling in the media and giving them interesting stories, or public protest. If there is cooperative motivation, one party does not have the goal of bragging about being the winner. Rather, the goal is proposals that both sides can point to as benefiting all parties and as giving attention to everyone's interests.

In accountability of process, negotiators have the responsibility of explaining what happened during discussions with counterparts. The people to whom they must explain the process are their constituents. If people know they will be accountable, they are motivated to examine issues under discussion from multiple perspectives. They know they will have to stand up in front of their constituents and answer sharp questions such as, "Is the other party fully committed to following through on its concessions related to the money issues?" Finally, time can be employed to the advantage of the negotiating parties. Mild rather than intense time pressures have advantages. If deadlines for a decision allow little time for negotiations, then there will not be opportunities to do the hard work of addressing the many concerns of the different parties. But if no deadlines are set, discussions can continue to meander without any pressure to move people toward decisions about negotiated proposals of benefit to all.

The Confirmation Bias. Communication is not just a presentation of what people think, that is, their cognitions (Chapter 2). In addition, people have an emotional investment in their communications: They feel they are right, they want to protect a certain valued view of the world, and they feel that others should think the way they do. Everyone is subject to the possibility of what has been called the confirmation bias (Oswald & Grosjean, 2004).

People Focus on Facts and Emotions to Support Preconceived Positions

"This should be an interesting task," Cindy Tanaka said to herself. Cindy had been asked by the senior managers of her organization to join a panel of employees that would make recommendations regarding promotions. Cindy, a mortgage banker, had worked in the same organization for eight years. As a college student, she had taken an internship in the organization, performed well, and was hired as a full-time employee after graduation. Cindy knew that Herb Schumate would be one of the candidates she would be considering. Cindy had worked with Herb when she was an intern, but doubted that he remembered this fact. She did not have particularly fond memories. Cindy thought that Herb was demanding, condescending, and treated her as a menial laborer rather than as an intern who wanted professional experience.

Cindy told her immediate supervisor that she knew many of the candidates for promotion and had both positive and negative experiences with them. Perhaps she should turn down the invitation. Her supervisor told her, "Everyone on the panel whose members will make recommendations is familiar with the work of the candidates. Such knowledge is valuable. The executives want to receive the recommendations of people who know the candidates well and who have observed their work for many years."

When the panel met, Cindy reviewed Herb's application. She found that she could not become impressed. Herb seemed to do work that was of average quality and which rarely went beyond the written requirements of his job description. His letters of recommendation seemed tame, with phrases such as "performs at a level comparable to people in his department with the same amount of education and job experience." When she discussed her observations with those of other panel members, however, she found that she had a minority opinion. Most other panel members thought that Herb's application was well prepared and that he was a good candidate for promotion.

Cindy may have fallen victim to the confirmation bias (Oswald & Grosjean, 2004). When people have strong preconceived views, they search available facts for evidence that supports these views. Since most collections of facts are not perfectly clear and are open to various interpretations, people can almost always find information to support the views that they already have formed. Examples can be seen during political campaigns. A Republican candidate makes a speech that targets wasteful spending on government programs for working-class families. Staunch Democrats complain that the candidate is trying to eliminate reasonable entitlements. Supportive Republicans applaud the same speech as advocating individual initiative and as getting the government off the backs of the electorate (Sherif et al., 1965).

In Cindy's case, memories of Herb's behavior during her internship eight years ago led to a predetermined opinion. She does not care for Herb and finds reasons to oppose his promotion application. She reviews work and concludes that it is of average quality, not realizing that this judgment is colored by her previous negative experiences. She does not stop to consider that her problems may have been due to a personality clash with Herb that rarely occurs with other employees. She interprets phrases comparing him as similar to others as indicative of mediocre work. But such a conclusion could indicate exemplary performance if Herb is a member of a highly productive department where the average measurable output is higher than similar departments in other organizations.

The confirmation bias is difficult to counter. Cindy can make attempts only if she is aware of it and consciously takes steps to challenge her preconceived views. If she is unable to do this by herself, she can benefit from listening closely to panel members who disagree with her. Realizing the existence of this bias, people who might be targets can supply information that is objective and that is less susceptible to varying interpretations. In

Herb's case, for example, he could submit specific data on his performance including reports about money brought into the organization, ratings of customer satisfaction, and number of requests received from coworkers that requested his collaboration on various projects.

The Self-Serving Bias. Another imperfection that occurs when people communicate stems from the need to present oneself as a decent, valued person who is worthy of attention. People are very skillful when examining the social situations in which they interact with others. They are adept at discovering current norms regarding what respected and high-status people do to acquire and to maintain their status (Buss, 2008). In situations where people can inflate their abilities and accomplishments, there is a great temptation to do so. This self-serving bias (Miller & Ross, 1975) is part of answers to the complex question, "Are we busier and working harder today than we were in previous decades?" Answers are also due to imperfections in memories: People simply cannot remember everything that happens to them. Self-serving and memory imperfections can work together when people forget incidents that threaten their positive self-image.

Workers Not Necessarily 'Busier Than Before'

Going through her mail, Julia Kubota opened a letter with two tickets to a political fund-raiser that would be held in three weeks. "Just what I need," she complained. "Here's another request for my time. And from talking to others, it's not just me. People are so much busier, with more demands on their time, than in years past. No one seems to have leisure time during which they can do exactly what they want." Although complaints like Julia's are commonly heard, research by behavioral and social scientists indicates an opposite conclusion: Americans have more leisure time than they did 40 years ago.

The University of Maryland's John Robinson has been one of the most active researchers on people's use of time, and published the book *Time for Life* (Robinson & Godbey, 1999; Bianci, Robinson, & Milkie, 2006). One conclusion, based on his work and that of independent research teams, is that people say they are busier than in years past but in reality have more time for hobbies, relaxation, and interactions with friends. What could be causing the difference between people's feelings about how busy they are with the fact that their leisure time has increased?

One reason is the difference in how information behind the two conclusions—busier and more leisure—is gathered by researchers and processed by people who are asked about their time. Let's consider the use of time over the last two months. When people talk about their uses of time, they are recalling many events and are coming up with a conclusion based on their memories. So when they say, "I am busier than in years past," they are making a conclusion today based on memories of the last two months. But in the research of Robinson and his colleagues, conclusions are based on hour-by-hour diaries. People report what they have been doing each hour shortly after the events by recording them in their diaries. Some readers may be familiar with the diary method of data gathering. They may have been participants in radio-listening or television-viewing surveys. They report their use of radio and television by filling in a daily diary when memories are fresh. Often, diaries show more television viewing than retrospective reports a month or so after people actually sat down in front of their televisions.

People do not try to be deceitful when they recollect past behaviors. Memories are not perfect, and people simply forget events that did not make much of an impact. They may have watched reruns of *Friends* and *Seinfeld* a month ago, but they simply do not remember these behaviors when asked about television viewing four weeks later. The same imperfections of memory affect reports of various uses of people's time. People may have had three important meetings at work that lasted about an hour each. All these meetings could have involved the possibility of working with new clients whose business would increase company revenues. Further, if their meetings were successful, this fact would be taken into account during people's yearly workplace evaluations carried out by company executives. A month after such meetings, people are more likely to remember them than they are the informal party that involved watching a three-hour football game on television in the company of friends. Given their memories, they are likely to make a conclusion that they have been very busy. But if they keep hour-by-hour diaries, the time spent watching football is recorded.

Another reason, suggested to me by Robinson, involves the self-serving bias since reports of deep involvement with one's work is a status symbol. In the United States, much of people's social identity is based on the work they do. When meeting others for the first time, people are more likely to ask, "Where do you work?" than "How do you spend your leisure time?" Social status, then, is more related to reports of hours spent at work than hours spent in activities of people's own choosing.

There are other reasons for the interesting distinction between people's complaints about busy lives and the results of careful research. One might be called the "What counts as leisure time?" question. Let's use the example of political fund-raisers or welcoming receptions for new employees at work. These might be scheduled from 7:00 P.M. to 9:00 P.M. on a Thursday. Do people view these as work or as leisure? If they enjoy meeting and talking with different people, some of whom they may not have met before, then they might consider the evening activities as part of their leisure time. If they do not like such events and would rather spend time with family and friends, or use the time to read a mystery novel, then attendance at the fund-raisers and receptions would be considered work.

Another example is time for exercise. Compared to 40 years ago, people are much more concerned with their own responsibilities for their health. They have scheduled time for exercise. If they view a one-hour walk as work, then they will complain about another burden on their day. If they view exercise as fun and as an opportunity to socialize with others, then they will think about it as leisure. Still another reason for views about increasing work time is that many aspects of life have become more complex. If people want to watch a TV show, they have the opportunity to examine the offerings of more than 200 channels. Forty years ago, people had only three or four channels to choose from. For many people, it may seem like work to find a television show that they want to watch.

Or, consider children's sports. When I was a child, there was no organized soccer program in any of the three communities where I lived. Friends and I would kick a ball around in a park or vacant lot, but there was no adult supervision. Today, there are organized soccer leagues with uniforms, protective pads, practice schedules, team names, and formal games that require the participation of trained referees. If parents feel it is a burden to supervise their children's participation in organized sports, then they will view their contributions to the team as work and will remember it as such.

SENSITIVE COMMUNICATION TOPICS AND METHODS: CAREFULNESS IS NEEDED

Some issues that arise during the communication process are very sensitive and demand extreme care. Sometimes, the issues involve methods of communication, such as attempting to phrase messages in a humorous manner (Morreall, 1991) or with short and concise words that communicators think will be understood (Gudykunst, 1983). Other issues stem from the sensitivity of the topic, as with male-female interactions (Buss, 2008; Tannen, 1990).

Humor: It Can Fall Flat. Has any reader ever met anyone who doesn't claim to have a great sense of humor? If the people do have such claims, they often fail in their attempts to communicate using humor.

Beware of People Who Think that They Are Humorous

The company for which Sarah Tatsuno worked had a policy of hiring people into jobs with a one-year probationary period. Any time within employees' first year, management could terminate them without concerns about legal recourse. After the first year, employees had more rights and could only be terminated after complex "for cause" hearings. After nine months, Sarah had an appointment with her boss, Janet Chung, and the agenda included a review of Sarah's job performance. Sarah thought that she had done well. She had brought in a great deal of business to her company, had represented the company at professional meetings, and interacted well with coworkers.

Janet was a person who thought she had a great sense of humor. She would tell jokes at company meetings and people would laugh politely. She interpreted the laughter as a sign that she should continue to be humorous. Janet thought a great deal of Sarah's work and looked forward to the meeting since the feedback about Sarah's first nine months would be positive. Trying to be light and witty, Janet used a light-hearted tone when saying, "I think that you are making progress toward the possibility of being hired for the second year." Sarah did not take this feedback well and wondered if she should seek a job elsewhere.

Janet was trying to use humor as a communication tool (Morreall, 1991), but she slipped on a banana peel. Humor is most effective when all parties know that fun and laughter are the goals of people's activities. When we watch *The Tonight Show*, we expect Jay Leno to tell jokes rather than give a lecture on the problems of the underclass. When we attend informal gatherings with friends on a Saturday evening, we know that there will be lighthearted banter. But when we meet with our bosses about performance evaluations, there may be a problem if the people involved have different expectations. If Sarah knew that Janet used humor as a way of communicating her positive attitudes about others, then the meeting might have been a success. But after only nine months in the organization, Sarah might not have known this aspect of Janet's approach to meetings. Without a shared framework for performance evaluations and accurate expectations about behavior during the meeting, there is the danger of miscommunication. This was certainly the case in the meeting between Sarah and Janet.

Another problem with Janet's behavior is that she mishandled a key aspect of humor. Funny stories involve two or more concepts that are twisted and manipulated in a novel manner (Attardo, 1997). People listening to jokes experience a sense of discovery when they figure out the twist and then experience the pleasure that accompanies laughter. Consider this workplace example: A reporter tells the city editor, "The baggage handlers at the airport staged a work slowdown as a protest against management." The editor replies, "How could anybody tell?" The two concepts being twisted are work slowdowns and the time it usually takes for people to receive their luggage while waiting at the carousels. Hasn't everyone noticed that their bags always seem to be the last ones to arrive? The reporter is likely to recognize the juxtaposition of the two concepts and might find the editor's comment humorous. In the case involving Sarah and Janet, however, two concepts that could form the basis for humor are not clear. Janet's lame combination of her positive attitude about Sarah and her actual comment are not likely to be appreciated by listeners.

Short, Terse Communication Codes. When people know each other well, they often use very short, concise phrases that are meant to communicate a great deal of information (Bernstein, 1971; Gudykunst, 1983). The use of such a communication style, sometimes called a restricted code, often occurs when people share the same cultural background, are close to each other in age, and have similar amounts of education. Problems arise when outsiders misinterpret these terse codes.

An Expansive Conversational Style Brings Advantages

My nephew recently called me from the mainland. He recently graduated from college and is seeking a job. He asked for my advice regarding his behavior during job interviews. I gave him several pointers. Job applicants should do extensive research on the companies where they want to interview. This can be done with the help of the Internet as most companies have Web sites and links to other helpful information. With the results of their research, job applicants do not have to ask basic information from members of the interview panel. Rather, they can ask more sophisticated questions and thus impress panel members with their knowledge and willingness to prepare for serious interviews.

I also gave him advice on communication style during interviews. I have observed him speaking with age peers in the monosyllabic code that young adults often use. They feel that a great deal of information is communicated through use of terms such as *hey, rad, cool, stoked,* and *bro.* But members of interview panels do not care for monosyllabic answers to their questions. They are looking for people who have good command of their mother tongue and who can give expansive answers showing their knowledge and ability to think clearly. Use of expansive language also shows that job seekers are comfortable meeting new people and explaining themselves to others.

Right after giving this advice, I received a copy of Jane Hyun's (2005) book, *Breaking the Bamboo Ceiling.* She addresses the issues facing Asian Americans as they interview, start their careers, and climb the ladder of success. One of the points she makes is that Asian Americans are not expansive when talking about themselves. Part of their socialization is to be modest when discussing their abilities. When good things are to be said, someone from a person's extended family is supposed to take the role of informal cheerleader. A modest communication style may work well when Asian Americans stay in the communities where they were socialized and where potential employers know relatives who can speak for candidates. But as Hyun points out, a modest style does not work well when Asian Americans apply for jobs in communities where they are not well known and where they are expected to speak up for themselves.

Communication scholars study how people actually use language. There is a distinction between restricted and elaborated codes (Bernstein, 1971). Restricted codes consist of very short and precise statements whose meaning is well known among family members and friends. A short telephone message saying "surf's up" can indicate that people will be picked up shortly for a trip to a favorite surfing spot. But this meaning is shared only by people who know each other, who have previously discussed the same favorite surf spots, who know what time they will be picked up, and so forth.

Elaborated codes are necessary when people do not know each other and when they do not share past experiences with each other. People have to expand from the two-word statement, "surf's up." They have to explain why they are making this observation, whether or not there is any action that will follow, and what the time frame will be for the actions. When people speak only with others who are well known, they do not have to use elaborated codes. Only a few words are necessary. In fact, if people use more words than are necessary others might think that they are putting on airs or trying to sound smart.

During job interviews, elaborated codes are necessary since applicants and members of interview panels do not know each other and have not shared past experiences. Job seekers are well advised to practice an expansive style so that they can explain their education, past work experience, and future goals.

After giving my nephew advice on his communication style, he told me, "I know how to speak to people who are a lot older than I am." I was glad to hear this. It means he knows the differences between various communication styles and the ways in which they are appropriate for different social situations.

Male-Female Interactions. Males and females bring differences to the workplace and these often have major effects on communications among colleagues (Tannen, 1990). Aid in understanding some of these differences has been provided by research in evolutionary psychology. A short introduction to this research field is helpful.

In recent years, behavioral and social scientists have examined evolutionary theory for insights into human behavior (Buss, 2008). This work is controversial, as shown by the number of school districts where the study of evolution is restricted. I am contributing to the controversy by suggesting that insights from the study of evolution can be applied to the study of everyday behaviors in the workplace. One of the basic assumptions in evolutionary theory is that our distant ancestors behaved in ways that increased the chances of their survival. If certain behaviors led to survival, then they became well established and passed on from generation to generation. Some of these behaviors became so privileged that people's brains developed to make their acquisition possible (Tooby & Cosmides, 2005). Examples are language learning, the startle reflex when there is danger nearby, and the ability to form alliances with others. Another example, with implications for today's workplaces, is the interaction of males and females.

For humans to survive into future generations, they must mate and have children. Men and women look for different features in potential mates (Buss, 2008). Men look for youth and physical attractiveness. Youth is central since there are limits to the childbearing years of women. Attractiveness is a sign that women are healthy, and so babies they bear may also be healthy. Women are looking for men with status and resources. They need men able to provide resources during the nine months of pregnancy, the pains of childbirth and its aftermath, and during the years necessary to raise children until they become self-sufficient. Men with high status titles and resources that can be exchanged for food and shelter are desirable.

In today's world, remnants of this age-old exchange of youth and attractiveness lead to frequently seen behaviors. Women dress and make themselves up to be attractive to members of the opposite sex. Men learn to present themselves in ways that emphasize their status and earnings potential. They may drive expensive cars, for example, to persuade women that they have a great deal of money. Some behaviors border on the inappropriate. Imagine a social gathering at the office that takes place at 5:00 P.M. on a Friday. The purpose of the gathering is to welcome the new company vice president. There are about 100 people present, some of them young and attractive and others who are older and well established in their careers. Who will, perhaps inappropriately, focus their attentions on young and attractive people so that they can improve their social lives? Men are more likely than women to turn the gathering into opportunities for dating.

Who will focus their attentions on older and well-established people who might have favors to distribute? Women are more likely to turn the gathering into opportunities to increase their resources in the forms of improved professional networks, information about promotions, and the development of political alliances in the workplace. This quest for favors is one reason older executives learn to dislike company parties. They complain that they came to have a good time, but instead they are hustled for favors.

These tendencies are subject to cultural changes. Given recent work-place policies concerning sexual harassment, men have to be careful about their interactions with females. And given that women can now earn large salaries and can hold down high-status jobs, they do not always need to be dependent on men for resources.

THE INFLUENCE OF THE SOCIAL SITUATIONS IN WHICH PEOPLE FIND THEMSELVES

People can learn to be very skillful at reading cues from the social situa-tions in which they interact with others (Blass, 2004; Dierdorff, Rubin, & Morgeson, 2009; Zimbardo, 2007). People are at a meeting in their organi-zation. Should they speak up if they disagree with what is being dis-cussed, or has a decision already been made regarding the issue under discussion? The boss weighs in with her opinion. Is it wise to disagree with her in a public forum, or would it be better to wait and to speak pri-vately with her in her office? An announcement has been made concerning a promotion possibility. Five people currently working in the organization can apply, and a headhunter has been hired to identity candidates cur-rently working in other organizations. Should the inside candidates apply, or do cues suggest that an outsider will be given preference?

The ability to read situational cues is part of people's innate abilities from their evolutionary heritage (discussed previously in this chapter). Our distant ancestors had to read cues in the situations where they found themselves, and their decisions had an impact on their survival (Buss, 2008). Should we stay in this current spot where we have been hunting and gathering, or should we move to another place that possi-bly has more abundant resources? Should we approach the strangers whom we see on the horizon, or should we be more wary since they might be bringing danger? Should we support candidate A or candi-date B in their quest to be leader of our group given the abilities the candidates have that can bring valuable resources to the group?

This emphasis on interpreting cues from social situations provides a major counterpoint to one of the most widely accepted myths about human behavior: People are consistent in their actions no matter where they find themselves. Specific examples are that assertive people are always likely to speak out in public, and that altruistic people will always volunteer for community service activities. The facts are that people are extremely sensitive to the social situations in which they find themselves and make adjustments in their everyday behaviors (Dierdorff et al., 2009; Zimbardo, 2007).

People who are very confident about their public speaking skills, and who are known to be good leaders, may be relatively quiet in cer-tain social situations. They may be at meetings with younger colleagues who need more first-hand experience in communicating their points. The leaders may decide to remain silent and let the younger employees make presentations and field questions. Leaders know that if they are the only attendees at the meeting who speak up, subordinates will not develop their skills. Or, confident and knowledgeable people may defer to someone with recognized credentials. I was involved recently in a project where one person formulated specific goals and acquired the necessary funding to carry out his plans. Twelve highly verbal individuals deferred to this person. They accepted his leadership because they felt he had the responsibility of communicating his wishes to those who agreed to help him with the project.

The fact that people can adjust to various social situations explains why they can accomplish so much. They can achieve various goals because they are able to behave in a variety of ways at different times. During the same day people can make sales calls, give constructive feedback to a subordinate, attend a Bible study group, and discuss algebra homework with their teenage children. They behave differently and in doing so demonstrate the range of human potential.

Making Adjustments to Bad Situations. Unfortunately, situations can be bad and many people adjust to them. Bad situations suck in good people and encourage them to engage in behaviors that are ethically troublesome (Blass, 2004; Zimbardo, 2007). In many communities, for example, there has long been the practice of giving campaign donations in the hopes of receiving government contracts at a later date. Further, people are supposed to accept the absurdity that engineers and architects give to campaigns and expect nothing in return. This is a bad situation. Good people, both donors and politicians, are stuck in a situation that draws out the worst in them.

One of many signs that people are facing bad situations is that there is a special language that people use to discuss their behavior. In the campaign contribution case, phrases like "we have always done it this way" or "we can bundle money from different employees and relatives" are used. At times, the communication is nonverbal. Politicians don't explicitly say that government contracts will be forthcoming. But the smiles, winks, and nudges people share communicate the same message.

Leaders can take steps to make bad situations better. They can examine common situations that people face and ask themselves, "Are there changes that can be made that will bring out the best in people rather than encourage their worst behavior?"

Mistaking Personality Traits for Situational Influences. Another way to understand the important topic of situational influences is to discuss a common mistake people make during their everyday lives.

When people observe the behavior of others, there is a strong tendency to make judgments about their personality traits (Tetlock, 1985). An individual who shows up late is seen as careless. The people making these judgments, also called attributions, do not take situational influences into account. Perhaps the individual is having car trouble or had to take care of a sick child. Or, an individual who turns down social invitations is seen as a loner. Situational influences may include the fact that the individual has to work on weekends to meet a work deadline, or is holding down a second job to make ends meet.

One reason why observers ignore situational influences is that they are often invisible. We can see individuals who come in late or who turn down social invitations, but we can't see the complex situational forces that are contributing to their behavior. Another reason is that it is more difficult to talk about situations because there is not a precise set of terms to describe them. There is a commonly used language to talk about personalities, and we use it often when referring to hard workers or to altruistic people. But there is not a widely used language to summarize the situational pressures everyone faces on a daily basis.

At times, situations can be bad and can bring out the worst in people. Consider donations to campaign contributions. Decent and well-meaning politicians and contributors are stuck in a system that leads to ethically troublesome behavior such as preferential treatment in the awarding of government contracts. Another bad situation occurs when there is an already-selected individual for a job that is widely advertised and for which many people apply. The selected person may be someone who is already well known to the hiring committee because of shared networks and community activities. But laws require that many jobs must be advertised widely, and so members of the hiring committee must go through the charade of carrying out an open search. People applying for the job must go through the time and expense of submitting their resumes and writing cover letters, unaware that their efforts are wasted.

An organization's leaders can improve bad situations. One way is to identify them. Bad situations are often marked by a language that is shared among a select group of people. Phrases such as "there is no other way to do it," or "let's not be too public about this" are giveaways. Another way is to constantly put oneself in the role of various people in different social situations. Questions such as, "How would I feel if I applied for a job that had already been filled by a favored candidate?" are appropriate. Still another way is to invite outsiders to observe various social situations and to make constructive comments. Many times, people become so wrapped up in their work that they fail to see alternative ways of behaving. Outsiders can offer valuable perspectives. In one of the best-known research studies of good people in bad situations, well-adjusted college students were assigned to roles in a simulated prison. Students given the role of guards became abusive, and students acting as prisoners became passive and accepting of their fate. The research, known as the Stanford Prison study (Zimbardo, 2007), was scheduled for two weeks but had to be terminated after six days because people's behavior became so outrageous. An outsider who visited the prison contributed to the decision to terminate. She reacted negatively to the behavior she observed, and in so doing forced the researchers to examine the implications of their work.

MODERN COMMUNICATION TOOLS: E-MAIL

In writing this chapter on communication, I find that I am drawing on research and commentary that concerns that entire span of human existence. I have made reference to our distant evolutionary past and the implications this has for today's communication practices (Buss, 2008; Tooby & Cosmides, 2005). There are other communication practices that were undreamed of by members of the previous generation, never mind our distant ancestors. One set of communication practices centers around the development and uses of e-mail (Gellenberg, 2009; Wells & Meche, 1999). Some readers will remember the earliest days of e-mail and will remember how norms have changed regarding its use.

Many of the early suggestions for appropriate e-mail use reminded me of what unruly students in a cooking class might do. The image that went through my mind was that the students combined flour and water, kneaded the resulting dough, and then threw it against the wall. Some of the dough would stick, and some would fall to the floor. The development of e-mail norms went through a similar process. Guidelines for appropriate behavior were suggested and tried out. Some stuck and became part of everyday e-mail use, and some suggestions fell by the wayside.

Early suggestions were that e-mail messages should be quick and informal. People were told that they should not worry about niceties such as punctuation, spelling, and capitalization of proper names. One reason for this suggested set of norms regarding informality was that e-mail was originally viewed as a supplement to old-fashioned mail with its elements of stationery, envelopes, and stamps. The thought that e-mail would merely be a supplement did not have a long shelf life. By the mid-1990s, many people were carrying out the majority of their correspondence through cyberspace. I first realized that I was not receiving much traditional mail when I was no longer able to collect postage stamps for one of my mentors. During the 1970s and 1980s, I could send him a package filled with international stamps approximately once every six months. Since 1995, I have been able to do this about once every two years.

With the increasing use of e-mail, norms became more formal. Recipients of e-mail would have no other impression of senders than the content of the messages. As a result, senders realized that to make a good impression (Grant & Mayer, 2009; Tetlock, 1985) they had to be careful. Positive impressions include coming across as well educated, articulate, and conscientious. This meant that the dreaded rules from people's elementary and high school educations had to be dusted off. Good spelling became important, especially as they learned that different recipients had "pet peeves" concerning the spelling of certain words. Similar care had to be put into issues such as capitalization, subject-verb agreement, punctuation, and vocabulary.

As software technology for e-mail improved, other considerations demanded attention. The forwarding of messages is very easy. So if people write a message, they have to be prepared for the fact that it can be forwarded to dozens if not hundreds of others (Gelenberg, 2009). Almost everyone I know has been caught in a "forward to many others" embarrassment. They criticized some people in an e-mail message and used colorful language while doing so. The people being criticized had the message forwarded to them and were not appreciative of the sentiments expressed. Or, a message sender had the intention of saying something positive about other individuals. But because the original message was not well constructed and could be read in different ways, people receiving the forwarded communication interpreted it in the most negative way possible.

Another feature of e-mail that can work against senders is that it is so fast. If people receive a message that stimulates negative emotions, they can write an angry reply and send it out before they have a chance to calm down. This has led to a good piece of advice that bosses now share with subordinates. On receipt of a message that might lead to an angry response, wait a day. Then, reread the message carefully. The original negative emotion may have been due to a careless initial reading. Even if a firm and somewhat unfriendly response is appropriate, people will be able to formulate their message in a more socially skilled manner (Baumeister, 2005) if they wait until they have better control of their emotions.

Another important aspect of e-mail is its ubiquity. Thirty years ago, e-mail was an informal tool for quick messages and exchanges of information among a small and highly computer-literate population. Today, virtually everyone is expected to have an e-mail address and e-mail often substitutes for yesterday's formal communications through stationery, envelopes, stamps, and post office workers who brave the possibility of barking dogs. The speed of communication through cyberspace is a great blessing. People receive an invitation to an important meeting that is sent through the use of a distribution list composed of 20 people. Twenty years ago, invitations to a similar meeting would have required 20 letters or phone calls. Today, messages can be sent to a distribution list in less than a minute. Recipients can type, "I can come," press "return," and let people know of their plans in fewer than 10 seconds.

In addition to its benefits, the convenience and speed of e-mail also has a downside. People can write messages and send them so quickly that they sometimes do not invest an appropriate amount of time in assuring message clarity. Further, message senders often forget that they make an impression on recipients. Carelessly worded messages, full of grammatical errors and misspellings, may lead recipients to conclude that the sender is poorly educated, ignorant, or both.

Another problem is that since e-mail has developed as a major communication tool in a short amount of time, norms for proper use are not well established (Gelenberg, 2009). The writers of etiquette books have spent decades developing norms for traditional stationery and envelope communications. These include norms for salutations that depend on how well the sender knows the receiver. The norms also include appropriate introductory sentences, phrases that are wise to avoid in letters meant to be cordial, and suitable closings.

E-mail has been in common use for about 20 years, and etiquette writers have not yet had the opportunity to vet various phrases that have become commonplace. As a result, senders can irritate recipients by using certain phrases that not all people consider appropriate and polite. One such phrase occurs after people send an e-mail requesting help from a recipient. The request might be to send some materials, fill out a questionnaire, or provide information on job openings. Senders sometimes use the phrase, "Thanking you in advance, I look forward to receiving your response." I find use of this phrase rude. If someone takes the time to respond to an e-mail with materials or information, then they deserve to be thanked after they perform these favors.

People sometimes use another phrase I dislike when they want detailed information about an issue. They e-mail me, "I will be in Honolulu next week and I would like to meet and to pick your brain." This phrase comes across as indicative of a callous person and as typical of someone who wants to exploit others. Fund-raisers do not e-mail wealthy people and say, "I'd like to meet and get a lot of money from you." People want to feel that they consist of more than their money and their information, just as physically attractive people want to be perceived as having assets other than their good looks. People with information are often willing to share it with others, but they do not want to feel exploited while doing so.

There are a few norms for e-mail use that have become more formal for some people but that have remained informal for others. For some unknown reason, people once were told to be highly informal when greeting others in the first line of their messages. Even if a sender was unknown to the recipient, a salutation such as "Hi Betty" was considered appropriate. Given that e-mail messages today may be a person's only contact with recipients, a retreat to etiquette books for proper ways of addressing others who are not close acquaintances is wise.

6

Ways of Increasing Effective Communication

CONCEPTS THAT ASSIST IN ATTEMPTS TO COMMUNICATE EFFECTIVELY

A reasonable conclusion from the previous chapter is that there are many potential sources of error when people make attempts to communicate with others, and there are errors when listeners attempt to interpret people's communications. This chapter continues this discussion, with more emphasis placed on ways of increasing the probability of successful attempts to communicate. I would like to start by discussing four concepts that, if understood, should assist in attempts to communicate. These concepts are especially helpful in understanding communication across various types of differences, such as those stemming from cultural background, age, gender, life experiences, and social class. The four concepts are high- and low-context (Gudykunst, 1983; Hall, 1959; 1966), verbal contrasted with nonverbal communication (Jandt, 1998; Mehrabian, 1968; Molinsky, Krabbenhoft, Ambady, & Choi, 2005), voice tone (Nakano, 2006), and reacting to negativity in communications (Foa & Chemers, 1967; Kaushal & Kwantes, 2006).

High- and Low-Context Communications. One of the themes that will be discussed in various chapters of this book is that people must be sensitive to the situational cues that surround them in their workplaces.

This type of sensitivity is central to understanding high- and low-context communications (Hall, 1959).

Shared Background Influences Expectations about Communications

At a meeting that took place in a Honolulu bank, Frank Jordan presented his business plan for a company that would link Hawaiian products to Asian markets. Frank had recently moved to Hawaii from Chicago. The others at the meeting were bankers and investors, all of whom had lived in Hawaii for most of their professional lives. Just as Frank was wrapping up his presentation, two of the most respected people at the meeting glanced at each other and exchanged nearly imperceptible nods. The loan officer who arranged the meeting noticed the gestures and called for a recess. Frank did not understand what was going on and wondered if his presentation had been poorly received.

Frank has encountered the distinction between high- and low-context communication. In places where people have known each other for long periods of time, communication is often high-context. This means that people do not have to use a large number of words to deliver their message. The content of the message is heavily influenced by various contextual cues. The two local businesspeople at the meeting knew each other well. They may have wanted to speak to each other before questioning Frank at the end of his presentation. The two may have wanted to make sure that "they were on the same page" during their responses to Frank's proposal. So they exchanged slight nods of the head. The loan officer, also from Hawaii, noticed the nonverbal exchange and suggested a recess.

In cultures where people often move from community to community, these subtle communication norms are less likely to be prominent (Molinsky et al., 2005). People do not know each other well, and so they are much more dependent on the exact words they choose to use while communicating. If Frank presented his business plan in a low-context culture, the businesspeople would be much more overt about their desire for a recess. One might say, "I would like to take a break to discuss one aspect of your proposal with my colleague. I think we will be able to ask more pertinent questions if we compare notes at this time."

In high-context communication, people know the meaning of messages without the need for extensive discussion. In low-context communication, people have to talk, discuss, and engage in give-and-take dialogue (Hall, 1959). Another example may be helpful. When my parents married in 1938, where would they live? Because they grew up

10 miles from each other in two small Vermont towns, they shared cultural expectations. The answer was that they would live where my father got a good job. They did not have to spend time discussing the question. Today, the question becomes part of low-context communication. People do not always share the same expectations. The man and woman have to consider the question carefully and discuss it extensively. They may decide to live where the woman has the best job prospects and promotion opportunities. The old high-context answer that centers on the male's career goals is no longer automatic (Hofstede, 2001).

Nonverbal in Addition to Verbal Content in Communications. One aspect of high-context communications is the use of nonverbal cues. After having attended a welcoming reception for a new company vice president for three hours, people who have been married for 15 years can glance at each other and determine if one or both wants to leave. The two people are interpreting very subtle nonverbal cues, and these are part of the context surrounding the goals they have when communicating with each other.

Messages Have Both Verbal and Nonverbal Components

The company at which Steve Atkins worked put out an announcement concerning the search for a new district manager. Steve learned that both internal candidates and outsiders to the organization could apply. He updated his resume, contacted people for letters of recommendation, and wrote a cover letter matching his qualifications and achievements to the job requirements listed in the announcement. Steve knew that these formal steps would not be enough and that he should also talk to the people responsible for the final decision concerning the district manager position. He asked for a meeting with his direct supervisor, Nancy Miyamoto, to tell her of his plans. Steve knew that Nancy would be contacted for a reference and so he wanted her support. After the meeting, one of Steve's friends asked, "How did your talk with your boss go?" Steve replied, "She used the right words indicating that she supported me, but I'm not sure about the rest of her message."

In thinking about his meeting with Nancy, Steve is being sensitive to both the verbal and the nonverbal aspects of their communication. Verbal aspects center on the choice of vocabulary words. Nonverbal aspects include important elements such as tone of voice, body movements, gestures such as rising when a person enters an office in contrast to remaining seated, and facial movements (Hinde, 1972). Estimates differ concerning how much of the total meaning of face-to-face communication is determined by verbal compared to nonverbal signals. Various additional factors will be influential, such as people's personalities and organizational norms. But it is safe to say that in many individual conversations, as much as 80 percent of the communicator's intent and the recipient's interpretation can be determined by nonverbal cues (Mehrabian, 1968).

For example, Nancy might choose to use the words, "I think that is a great idea," when Steve talks about his plans to apply for the district manager. This could be very positive if Nancy uses an animated tone of voice, smiles when talking, maintains eye contact, and shows a relaxed body posture. But the message could be very negative if Nancy uses a snide tone of voice, frowns and looks up at the ceiling when talking, and shows a tense body posture. Nancy can also use a neutral set of nonverbal behaviors to accompany her choice of vocabulary. Her tone of voice can be rather flat, neither effervescent nor snide. She can maintain eye contact, but speak with a slight rather than glowing smile. Nancy might choose to communicate this way if there is another candidate besides Steve who has asked her for a recommendation. She may want to be supportive of both candidates and not communicate a preference for one over the other.

The combination of verbal and nonverbal cues is complex and no one is accurate all the time when sending or receiving messages. One way of increasing accuracy is for people to be sensitive to each other's baselines. People develop habitual ways of behaving, and if they behave in a similar manner on different days, these are known as their baselines. Some people are constantly excited and animated and so it can be hard to determine when they are truly in favor of a workplace proposal. Some people are very cool and calm, and so it can be easier to interpret nonverbal cues indicating a positive reaction. A slight grin from one person may be the equivalent to the beaming smile from another. A move from a poker face to clear distress from one person may be equivalent to the slight frown shown by another person.

Voice Tone and a Soft Communication Style. The tone that people use when communicating with others was referred to when Nancy used the phrase, "I think that is a great idea." Many times, people can use a certain vocabulary that might be offensive to others. But if they are sensitive to the social context in which the term is used, and use the appropriate tone of voice, then they can meet their communication goals (Haskard, Williams, DiMatteo, Heritage, & Rosenthal, 2008). Several of the examples, below, are from my experiences living in Hawaii.

The use of nonverbal cues such as voice tone is especially important in cultures that have a strong oral tradition. In such cultures, written language is a relatively new introduction. People still talk to each other a great deal and have not always adopted conventions based on written communications. In Hawaii, there are still reminders that oral traditions are much older than written communications. Many people still prefer face-to-face interactions with others (Brislin, 1981) rather than communications through letters or phone calls. This can be seen in the local tradition of responding to invitations to social gatherings. Even if the hosts of such gatherings put "RSVP" at the bottom of invitations, they should not expect that all people will respond with a note or phone call. Rather, the invitees feel that they may see the host at the beach or at the shopping center. Then, they can tell the host that they would like to come to the gathering.

The importance of nonverbal cues during oral communications has to be kept in mind when ethnic group epithets are used. Many people from the mainland United States find the word *haole* to be offensive. The term roughly translates as "outsider," and it is well enough known to be the answer to the clue "foreigner in Hawaii" in the *New York Times* crossword puzzle. Realizing that the term most often refers to Anglos from the mainland United States, targets of the term feel that its use reduces them to a negative stereotype and that users of the term would be offended if epithets for their own groups were used in the same way. In the workplace, employees are filing complaints that the use of ethnic group epithets contributes to a hostile environment that leads to lower worker productivity.

Epithets to describe ethnic groups are used more frequently in oral than in written communications. Given the choice of vocabulary during face-to-face communications, nonverbal cues must be integrated into the task of message interpretation. The tone of voice used when *haole* is used needs special attention. When the term is used with a pleasant tone of voice, the term can be descriptive rather than evaluative. That is, speakers might use the term to describe someone and to distinguish that person from others. "Let's ask the *haole* girl to be on our company volleyball team" can simply refer to a person who played well during a picnic at the beach last weekend.

When the term is used with a negative tone, then it probably will be interpreted as evaluative. If people say "the *haole* guy who was the first to speak at the union meeting" with a sneer in their voices, they are probably referring to a shared negative stereotype. These can include the perceptions that mainland Anglos always have opinions about which they are extremely confident, speak in a very loud voice, and think they know how to run things after living in Hawaii for a few months.

The need to interpret cues beyond the choice of vocabulary needs to be applied to all ethnic group epithets. When my children were younger, I was involved as a coach in various youth athletic leagues.

At basketball tryouts, a coach said that he would like to work with "the *Portagee* kid" (a local term in Hawaii for people with Portuguese ancestry). While some listeners may have found the term offensive, I did not. He was trying to distinguish among the basketball hopefuls who were displaying their talents, and he clearly had admiration in his voice for one youngster's dribbling, passing, and rebounding skills.

A nonjudgmental tone of voice, then, can contribute to communications that are meant to leave listeners with positive impressions of the speakers (Gibson, 2005). A nonjudgmental tone is part of what is sometimes referred to as a "soft style." Such a style includes a mild tone of voice, a willingness to listen respectfully to the views of others, and a willingness to be indirect when making suggestions. An example of a direct comment is, "We should add more radio advertisements to our marketing campaign." A softer, more indirect statement would be, "I wonder if we should consider adding more radio spots? What do you think?" The very direct statement aimed at another person, "You are absolutely wrong on this issue!" should be replaced. A softer alternative is, "I believe that there is another position on this issue that should be examined."

There is an interesting exception in Hawaii. Activists who advocate various political causes often shout at each other and pay little attention to the positions of those who disagree. I believe they would be more effective if they used a gentler tone of voice and engaged in more thoughtful listening.

I am quick to admit that a soft style is not effective everywhere. In other parts of the United States, especially in big cities, people often have to be much more vocal and direct or their views will be ignored during fast-moving meetings where everyone is trying to be heard (Milgram, 1970). People from Hawaii seeking jobs on the mainland are wise to talk to colleagues and friends who have lived elsewhere. Locals with ambitions for mainland jobs will find that practice sessions where they speak in a louder, more direct, and sometimes confrontational manner are valuable. One person with whom I have worked closely recently interviewed for jobs on the mainland as well as in New Zealand and Australia. He told me that the exchanges of questions and answers were much more intense and pointed than those to which he had become accustomed during his eight years in Hawaii.

Likewise, people from the mainland are wise to practice a gentle and indirect style (Nakano, 2006). Given the local preference for softer interactions, people from Hawaii are often uncomfortable with mainlanders who are quick to disagree and who are familiar with direct confrontation. Locals often have very thin skins since they have not frequently participated in the very direct give-and-take that is common in mainland conversations.

When I give talks to mainland businesspeople looking at opportunities in Hawaii, I often cover this point. I ask the mainlanders to think of people with whom they went to high school or college. I continue, "Think of people who were extremely thin skinned. You could not disagree about anything because they would take it personally (Pistole & Arricale, 2003). You could not criticize anything going on in your community because they would somehow feel that you are making negative references about them. What did you do to get along with these people? If you have such people in mind, treat everyone in Hawaii as if they were these people from your high school or college days."

Reacting to Negativity. Especially when they have ambitious work-related goals, people will receive negative reactions (Kaushal & Kwante, 2006). One reason is jealousy. Ambitious people may put others in a less favorable light. Another reason is that the thinking and reasoning behind people's ambitions may be unfamiliar to others. Rather than trying to say something positive about an idea that is unfamiliar, others are more likely to respond negatively or with a blank stare. This is common when people present their ideas for entrepreneurial ventures (Foo, Uy, & Baron, 2009).

Entrepreneurs Are Certain to Hear Discouraging Words

After working in a large hospital for three years, John Olsen examined where his life was going. Now 26 years old, John was a college graduate who majored in biology. In his selection of college electives, he had taken three courses in business and had also recently attended a night course titled "Writing a Business Plan." John thought a great deal about whether he should quit his current job and strike out on his own in an entrepreneurial venture. He did not particularly like his current work and could not see himself driving on the freeway to the same office for the next 20 years. In addition, he had little respect for his superior, who had few good ideas of his own and took credit for the work of his subordinates. John enjoyed the idea of being his own boss.

John had always been close to members of his extended family. He told people of his plans to quit his current job and to start a medical supplies company that would market to both physicians and their patients. He planned to give special attention to customers interested in alternative medicines. Many people questioned his decision. His father pointed to the statistics that indicated the percentage of start-up small businesses that fail. His aunt reminded him that his current job was very secure and that he currently did not have to worry about a regular paycheck. "There is no guarantee of a regular income when you start your own business," she continued.

People considering entrepreneurial ventures are almost certain to face discouraging comments from others (Foo et al., 2009). To be successful, entrepreneurs have to find a niche that is somewhat unfamiliar and does not bring immediate nods of recognition from people (Saviotti & Pyka, 2004). Given unfamiliarity with the entrepreneurs' ideas, friends and relatives cannot respond with positive comments about all the other people who have made money pursuing the niche. If large numbers of people had exploited the niche, then there would be less likelihood of new opportunities that could be pursued by an entrepreneur such as John. Entrepreneurs have to become accustomed to blank stares when they describe their ideas.

Entrepreneurs have to assume the role of nonconformists, and there will always be people who criticize individuals who are different. Negative comments will always be directed at individuals who want to pursue an unfamiliar lifestyle and who are willing to give up security for the uncertainty that always accompanies risk taking. Given this certainty, entrepreneurs might welcome discouraging comments. They can take this as a sign that they are pursuing an idea that others have not already exploited to the point where there are no more business opportunities.

Even though negative comments will be forthcoming, entrepreneurs are wise to think about them carefully. There may be some wisdom hidden in the feedback received from friends and relatives. Entrepreneurs are sometimes overly optimistic about the probability of their future successes. If they listen carefully to pessimistic feedback, they will be stimulated to engage in more careful thought. They will think more carefully about the importance of job security in their lives, the dread that may be forthcoming when money flow is uncertain, and the presence of various rival companies competing for customer allegiance. All these and other issues should be carefully considered by people who want to start new businesses.

OUTCOMES RESULTING FROM EFFECTIVE COMMUNICATION

Communication is not an end in itself. Rather, it is an important tool to be used in the quest for various company goals. All of us have been at meetings where people rambled on and on about inconsequential matters. This experience is captured by the common saying, "They seemed interested in hearing themselves talk." The goals under discussion are more central to organizational success than the self-enhancement that comes from talking loud and long. Four goals will be discussed here: organizational justice (Fischer, 2008), integrating expertise through participation (Locke & Latham, 1990), relationship building (Brewer, 2007; Brislin,

1981), and acting on rather than merely comprehending executive communications (Baumeister, Vohs, & Funder, 2007).

Organizational Justice. Issues of justice center on questions such as, "Are employees being treated fairly? If they have concerns, are there ways of voicing these without fear of reprimands? If they work hard, is it clear to them that they will be rewarded?" Different forms of communication assist executives in their goal of answering "yes" to these questions.

Outcome and Procedural Justice

After three years of hard work for his company, Dwight Turner felt that he deserved a raise. He prepared a list of his accomplishments and made an appointment with his boss, Karen Watanabe. Dwight felt that he had a good relationship with Karen, and he knew of her reputation as a fair-minded person. At the meeting, Dwight presented his case for a raise, and Karen listened carefully. She asked Dwight to expand on a few of his points. Dwight thought that the meeting went well. A week later Karen made an appointment with Dwight. She informed him that she could not give him a raise and then explained the reasons for her decision. Although disappointed that he would not receive a raise, Dwight did not become angry and did not start looking for a job at another company.

This incident deals with the distinction between outcome justice and procedural justice (Fischer, 2008; Greenberg, 1997). Dwight wants a certain outcome: a raise. Other outcomes people want in their workplaces include promotions, vacation time during certain months, better parking spaces, larger offices, and travel to professional conferences. Procedural justice refers to the policies set up by an organization and the attitudes of decision makers that allow fair consideration of employees' requests. Procedures should be clear concerning how raises can be requested and how people can apply for promotions and larger offices. Similarly, policies should be clear concerning who has access to desired parking spots and how decisions are made concerning vacation time and conference travel. Favored employees should not have an advantage simply because they know the arcane and under-communicated procedures for making requests. Most importantly, decision makers should communicate that they are unbiased and that they value all people who make requests. Decision makers should listen carefully, should show respect, and should not rush the person who is making the request. If decision makers frequently glance at their watches, this betrays their lack of interest in the employee.

Certainly outcome justice is important. All employees want their bosses to grant their requests. But employees know that resources are limited. They know that their companies cannot grant raises to everyone wanting them. They realize that there will be many people competing for a limited number of promotions. They know that there are limits to "perks" such as large offices, travel, and summer vacation time. But procedural justice is just as important (Greenberg, 1997). If bosses show respect for their employees and give them a fair hearing, then employees will often set aside their disappointments with outcomes. Bosses should also communicate the reasons for their decisions, and this is sometimes best handled after they make appointments at times convenient to the employees. Karen was wise to take this step as part of her procedural justice concerns.

The Development of Interpersonal Relationships. Humorous commentary among company employees and good-natured ribbing are not types of communication that should be eliminated in organizations (Morreall, 1991; Schnurr, 2009). Such communications can assist in the development of positive interpersonal relationships that can be called on when workloads increase suddenly due to issues such as market expansions and the introduction of new products and services.

Office Banter Can Prepare People for Serious Discussions

Three colleagues were having lunch in their company's cafeteria. Bob Perkins, Kimo Sumida, and Tom Chun had worked together for a year at the same investment firm in Honolulu. They began talking about sports.

> Kimo (to Bob): "I see that Utah State is going to the Copper Bowl this year. Didn't you go there for college?"
> Bob: "Yes, and I have the skiing injuries to prove it."
> Tom: "My fondest childhood memories are watching the Copper Bowl game on television with my father. We'd look forward to the game all year!"
> Kimo: "What will Utah State do with the proceeds from their Copper Bowl appearance? Will the football team upgrade from Motel Six to the Holiday Inn on their next road trip?"
> Bob: "I can see that you're working hard on your MBA degree with sophisticated financial analyses like that one!"

Later, a fourth colleague joined the group. Mary Stevens has a Deaf nephew and was taking sign language courses during her lunch hour at a nearby community college. Tom pointed to an empty seat and Mary sat down. Kimo began wiggling his fingers and waving his hands in an attempt to mimic sign language.

> Kimo (to Mary): "What did you learn to say today, Mary?"
> Mary: "I learned to say that I never see you surfing when the waves are higher than four feet!"

Bob: "With you knowledge of surfing, you could be an adviser to those movies they are making on the North Shore."

Mary: "Right, my start in show biz. I'll have to get your advice on investments when I enter the higher tax brackets."

Do conversations such as these serve any positive purpose in the workplace? I believe that the answer is "yes." This sort of bantering solidifies collegial relations among people (Schnurr, 2009). Participation in such conversations signals messages such as, "I am one of you and I am not putting myself above or below anyone." This bantering also shows that people have a sense of humor, and this can be a great asset in people's contributions to positive morale in their organizations.

Another benefit is that banter assists people in thickening up their skins. When people are so sensitive that offhand or humorous comments are always seen as personally insulting, they will find themselves cut off from informal conversations in an organization. As a result, they will find that they do not receive practice in the give-and-take of discussions during serious policy-making sessions at work. If they perceive any disagreements with their suggestions as personal attacks, they will not be effective participants in policy-making meetings. Participation in lunchtime banter can also provide practice for quick thinking. In the example, the four people's comments are droll rather than crude and involve clever thinking rather than appeals to the overused language of the gutter. Quick thinking "on one's feet" is a valuable contribution to bring to important workplace meetings (Griffin & Ouellett, 2007).

Employee Participation. The best executives realize that their major assets are the talents of their employees. It is the executives' responsibility to ensure that employees have opportunities to use their talents.

When I give workshops in organizations, I almost always touch on communication skills. I sometimes begin discussions by asking people about examples of good and poor communications. At one workshop a participant said, "Whenever I think about good communication skills in organizations, I think of managers who are able to obtain cooperation from workers. If workers are able to make contributions, this will improve the workplace in many ways. Workers will feel that their input is valued. Their contributions should improve the quality of a company's products and services. When their contributions are implemented, workers feel a sense of accomplishment. But not every manager is good at encouraging workers to participate. I admire those managers who can."

Encouraging participation from workers (Pencavel, 2003; Strauss, 2006) is based on a number of social skills. The first is the ability to make workers feel comfortable about speaking up and making suggestions. Many workers complain that, in the past, their contributions have been ignored. They carefully prepared some suggestions, made them known to management, and then heard nothing. As a result, they are hesitant to speak up when one of their current managers asks for suggestions about workplace improvement. Good managers, then, must communicate that suggestions are welcome. They must have developed an atmosphere of trust in their organizations so that workers are convinced they will not be punished if they make controversial suggestions. In addition, managers must follow through on the suggestions and either implement them or explain why the suggestions cannot be used at the present time. Workers prefer being told why a suggestion cannot be used to being told nothing at all.

If workers are highly resistant to making suggestions, good managers can engage in a series of steps that often lead to increases in idea sharing (Amy, 2008; Houston, Blankstein, Alan, & Cole, 2010). First, managers call workers together and ask them to discuss aspects of their jobs that seem to be going well. Most people are willing to discuss positive aspects of their work since they are not challenging authority and are not being asked to offer criticisms. After carefully listening to worker contributions, managers then must make the judgment about whether or not people seem comfortable with the group discussion format. If not, then other nonthreatening questions should be asked. One such question is, "Are there things that our competition is doing that seem to be successful for them?" Workers may be willing to discuss the competition's advertising or promotional campaigns without feeling that they are criticizing the management of their own organization.

Once managers make the judgment that workers are comfortable with this group participation, they can ask more difficult questions. One is, "What aspects of your current work are difficult?" After collecting answers, the next question can be, "What are ways of decreasing these difficulties and making things easier for you?" Answers to these questions should lead to the formation of goals (Locke & Latham, 1990) for workplace improvement and to ways of attaining these goals.

I have seen tremendous amounts of money wasted when managers bring in outside consultants who are supposed to make suggestions about improvement. Workers often know more about the details of making products and delivering services than do managers or hit-and-run consultants. When managers solicit and use suggestions provided by workers, they are taking advantage of expertise that is too often underutilized.

Acting on Employer Directives. Many times, executives will communicate their directives and will conclude that they have been effective. After a few months, however, they may find little evidence that anyone paid any attention to their directives. This is the theme of this critical incident.

Not All Communications from Executives to Employees Are Taken Seriously

"I try to communicate clearly with my employees, but sometimes I feel that I am not successful," Karen Fong told her executive assistant. Karen was president of a health maintenance organization. She had been on the job for six months, having taken over from a former president who had not been popular with doctors, nurses, and other staff members. In fact, the organization had the reputation of being tough on presidents, as four had come and gone over the last seven years.

One of Karen's goals was to decrease the number of complaints about health care services. She directed the manager of the human resources division to develop a system that would allow patients to give feedback about the quality of medical care they had received. She also asked the managers in accounting, custodial services, and information technology to prepare reports on different initiatives that she wanted to see implemented. Three months after communicating her directives, Karen was disappointed with the results. The department managers had given her plans for the implementation of various innovations, but she felt that they represented half-hearted efforts. She wondered if she could have been clearer in her communications.

Karen has encountered a common problem. Executives give directives, and little seems to happen. One reason for the problem is that employees try to determine the seriousness of the directives that executives order. Executives talk about many organizational issues, and employees have the task of sorting through the talk to determine the issues that require time and effort. I once worked for an organization that changed its accounting procedures every year. A new office manager came in with still another new set of procedures that were quite complex and difficult to learn. Employees complained, "Why should we learn this new system when it will probably be changed next year?" In Karen's case, her problem is compounded because so many presidents have come and gone. If employees do not like a directive, they can stall if they believe that the president will not be with the organization very long.

Executives will see more implementation of their directives if they are more careful in their communications. They should keep three concepts in mind: distinctiveness, consistency, and consensus (Kelley, 1967; 1972).

1. Distinctiveness means that executives must deliver messages that stand out from the everyday verbalizations. Messages must be

presented in a way that communicates a sense of importance. Executives should be careful when communicating high-priority directives. If they do not prioritize, employees will have a difficult time figuring out the difference between less and more important initiatives.

2. Consistency means that executives have to communicate the same message at different times, to different audiences, using various communication methods. They will have little success with their initiatives if they seem to be saying one thing when talking with doctors, another when talking with patient advocacy groups, and still another when talking with television reporters. Executives do not want to develop the reputation of having multiple faces depending on the type of audience they are addressing.

3. Consensus means that various people associated with the initiatives feel that they will improve the organization. Employees become confused when an executive issues a directive and mid-level managers seem unenthusiastic about it. Executives need to explain the reasons for their initiatives to their managers and ensure that everyone has bought into the planned changes.

Many times, managers will be able to suggest improvements to the executives' directives if they know the outcomes that are desired (Pencavel, 2003; Strauss, 2006). Managers are more likely to put time and effort into implementing the directives if their suggestions have been recognized. Executives will increase their chances of success if all their messages contribute to the same theme. If Karen wants to decrease the number of health maintenance organization member complaints, she should frame her directives in terms that will help in the implementation of this goal. With carefully constructed communications, Karen can communicate to employees in human resources, accounting, custodial services, and information technology how their efforts will lead to decreased complaints and increased member satisfaction.

When preparing her communications in this manner, Karen is keeping in mind the points of view of her employees. This ability to understand the viewpoints of others is a key to negotiation skills.

NEGOTIATION

What do the following terms have in common: negotiation, conversation, discussion, and talk story? All involve give-and-take between two people or among a larger number of people (De Dreu, 2005; Thompson, 1991). This give-and-take distinguishes these behaviors from the one-way communication that is typical of a sermon or a speech during which the speaker makes a set of demands. This distinction between two-way and one-way communication is frequently forgotten during interactions with others, especially when intense emotions begin to play a role (Hammer, 1997). Let's use an example involving a manager and her subordinates.

Successful Negotiations Require Respect for Others

Katie Percy supervises 12 scientists in the research-and-development department of a biotechnology company. She would like her subordinates to put more of their time into research on the treatment of genetic diseases in children. On the one hand, she could simply send out a memo to her employees requiring that they follow her directive. But she realizes that this might not be very effective. Employees in research and development are often very well educated, intelligent, and independent in their thinking. They do not react well to being told exactly what they should be doing in their choice of research projects. They react with more enthusiasm when asked about their opinions concerning the best projects for their future endeavors.

Realizing this, Katie calls her employees together for a meeting. She lists the reasons why she feels that workers should emphasize research on genetic diseases. Given that she realizes the scientists will have strong opinions, she listens carefully to their arguments. If she does this, she is beginning the process of negotiating. She knows that the scientists will have various concerns. They will want to know about the status of their current projects. They will want to know about start-up costs that will accompany a switch to more research on genetic diseases. They will want to examine their own education and work experience to determine if they have the expertise to make the move that Katie recommends. They will be concerned about how research according to Katie's preferences will affect their long-term career development.

Successful negotiations almost always depend on flexibility and a willingness to adjust one's preferences on hearing the positions put forward by others. Katie will have to bend a little to the preferences voiced by her scientists. For example, she may express a willingness to allow scientists to complete their current work. Or, she can fund attendance at professional conferences where the scientists can be exposed to current basic research related to genetic diseases. The key to negotiations is to recognize that other people have positions on important issues (Fisher & Ury, 1983). These others will want to see that attention has been given to their opinions, attitudes, and preferences.

Good negotiators demonstrate a willingness to listen to others and to incorporate their views into final plans for changes in organizational policy. Katie is likely to experience more success in negotiations if she does her own research and learns about employee concerns prior to calling them into a meeting. She can then address these concerns when she presents her position. The opposite of negotiation is a podium-pounding diatribe punctuated with a statement such as, "I demand that my position becomes adopted as the company policy!" Such statements are often delivered in a harsh, unpleasant, and insulting tone of voice. If people make demands, they are ignoring a basic principle of negotiations: Realize that others have positions that must be recognized and respected (Thompson, 1991).

Many times, people enter a meeting room with the goal of honest negotiations. However, this willingness changes as people share different opinions and express their disagreements. When faced with intense disagreements, many people become emotional and change their behavior from negotiation to making a set of demands. People who develop the reputation of good negotiators over a period of many years do not "lose their cool" when challenged, and instead maintain respect for others and their disagreements (Brislin, 1991).

Preparation for Negotiations. All efforts associated with negotiations do not take place in a room with others who have varying viewpoints. A great deal of the required effort takes place prior to formal negotiation sessions (Fisher & Ury, 1983). Good preparation for actual face-to-face negotiations is essential.

In Negotiations, Have Your Ducks Lined Up

After two years as middle managers at the same food-processing plant, Ken Johnson and Mike Yang felt that they should schedule a meeting with their boss to discuss adjustments to their salaries. Their supervisor was Kathy Inaba, who had been with the company for 15 years and who was known as a skilled negotiator. Executives often asked her to travel to the home offices of various suppliers to represent the organization in negotiations for the purchase of various supplies. Ken and Mike had scheduled meetings with Kathy that would take place on a Wednesday. Ken was to meet Kathy during the morning, Mike during the afternoon. On a Friday, five days before their meetings, Ken asked Mike if he would like to have a drink at about 5:00 P.M. Mike replied that he would be working late that evening to prepare for his meeting with Kathy. Ken responded, "I don't know why you need so much time to prepare. Kathy knows our work. We just go in there and tell her what we think we are worth."

Ken may find that he is underprepared for his meeting. Negotiations are not one-way communications during which one person makes demands or requests and the other person listens. Negotiations involve the give-and-take of suggestions and proposals. Mike is spending extra time preparing himself. Good preparation includes knowing what Kathy's positions are on a variety of company issues. How much money does she have in her budget for salary raises? What are new initiatives she thinks the company should undertake? How can her subordinates contribute to these initiatives? What has been Kathy's own salary history in the company? At what points over her 15 years did she receive raises?

If Mike knows the answers to these and other questions, he is in a much better position to negotiate with Kathy. He will be prepared to answer any queries that Kathy poses. If Kathy makes appeals to her limited budget, Mike can point to the possibility of shifting from other budget items that are of lower priority, given her plans for future initiatives. Kathy may argue that Mike is requesting a very large raise for someone who has been with the company for only two years. However, if he is well prepared, Mike can counter with statistics showing that he is requesting a raise that is consistent with that given to other productive employees who have worked for the company for a comparable number of years. He then has to back this claim up with a summary of his contributions to the company.

The wisdom of knowing what others are thinking and knowing what they desire is useful in all sorts of negotiations (Thompson, 1991). When buying a car, customers can negotiate a price with the salesman and with the sales supervisor. Customers should make a list of what features they want in a car. After deciding on two or three possibilities, they should find out how much dealers paid for the cars. This information is available on several Web sites. They should know what dealers can charge as a reasonable markup. Customers should be aware of features such as extended warranties that salespeople will propose and will claim are essential. With this information, customers will be prepared to agree on a reasonable price. They will also have reason to walk away from the negotiations if they feel that their well-prepared proposal for a price is not accepted by the car dealership.

Returning to the example of salary negotiations, Mike is likely to reap additional benefits, given his careful preparation. Kathy may appreciate his efforts and may be more likely to grant the raise. She may say to herself, "I think it's fine that Mike was well prepared and that he 'lined up his ducks.' He can bring this same talent for knowing the desires of others to his work in attracting new customers and clients to our company."

Compromise. There are many adages that help people remind themselves that compromise is necessary in negotiations (Brislin, 1991; Crick, 1982). "Half a loaf of bread is better than none" is probably the best known.

Successful Negotiations Involve Research and Compromise

As previously discussed, a key to good negotiations is to remember that there are more than two people involved and that everyone involved has concerns that they want to see addressed (Fisher & Ury, 1983). For example, several workers may meet and agree to file a grievance about an abusive boss, a mid-level manager in the company where they are employed. The company president, Dan Esposito, agrees to meet with the workers. The workers have clear concerns: They want their boss removed, reprimanded, or at least sent to a training program dealing with effective management and leadership. The workers will be much more effective in their negotiations if they keep in mind that the company president will also have concerns that he will want to see addressed.

Dan will want to be seen as someone who stands behind his managers. He will not want to be seen as someone who can be pushed around by the latest gripe that workers present to him. He will also not want to be seen as having made a mistake if he played a major role in the hiring of the manager who is now the target of the workers' anger. The workers will be much more effective if they are genuinely concerned with Dan's worries and with making Dan look good in the eyes of all company employees.

They can start with the request that their boss be fired, realizing that this is a start to the negotiations and that it will probably not be accepted. They can then listen carefully to Dan. They should not interrupt him and instead should listen respectfully. If they have done their homework—a step always recommended for good negotiators—there should be few surprises during Dan's presentation of his concerns, because the workers will be familiar with them. After listening to Dan, the workers should counter with a recommendation that clearly integrates aspects of his presentation. Negotiations can continue until a compromise agreement is reached that is satisfactory to all (Atran & Axelrod, 2008).

The final decision might be that Dan will meet with the manager to address the specific behaviors that the workers identified as abusive. If the manager does not improve within a month, based on reports from an already-scheduled follow-up meeting with the workers, Dan will send the manager to a training program for the development of human relations skills. With this compromise, both Dan and the workers have addressed some of the issues that they brought to the negotiations. They didn't get everything they wanted, but that is the nature of negotiations. People give a little here, take a little there, and hammer out an agreement that is satisfactory to all (Atran & Axelrod, 2008; Brislin, 1991).

So why don't people negotiate in this manner more often? One reason is that there is a great deal of work involved in determining the concerns of others who are part of the negotiation process. People may not be willing, or may not know how, to do the hard work of discovering the goals of others. Another reason is that it is a lot more fun to make a set of demands that take into account only the position of oneself, coworkers, and friends. It is enjoyable to make these demands in a loud voice and to engage in vigorous body movements while doing so.

After a speaker makes a set of such one-sided demands, there will usually be others who come up and offer enthusiastic congratulations and appreciation for "taking a stand against the powerholders." Speakers are congratulated far less often if they offer compromises that integrate the concerns of multiple parties in a negotiation. In fact, they might become the target of boos and hisses if they are seen as "not tough enough." Realizing this, parties in a negotiation often have to answer the question, "Do we want to be popular, or do we want to be effective negotiators who can develop workable solutions to problems?"

7

Understanding Power in the Workplace

INTRODUCTION

As introduced in Chapter 1, a major theme of this book is that people who understand workplace dynamics such as cognitive processes, group formation, communication, leadership development and other issues will have a greater chance of job satisfaction and life satisfaction. In my own personal experience, understanding power and its attractions to many people has been very important in my own efforts at workplace satisfaction. Power refers to influence in one's workplace and community, the ability to have one's preferences put into action, and the ability to help others with their work efforts in the expectations that these others will eventually return favors. If there is one substitute word for power, it is "clout" (Brislin, 1991; 2001).

Some young people have socialization experiences that lead to an understanding of power. They attend dinner parties with their lawyer fathers and politician mothers and keep up discussions with influential guests. They attend fund-raisers for political candidates, volunteer for community activities where they meet movers and shakers, and become comfortable interacting with school peers when they have titles such as "student body president." I had few such childhood experiences and so had to play "catch up" when I was well past 30 years old.

One personal experience may be instructive. I once worked for an organization where employees submitted proposals, and after a review some of the proposals would be funded. Decision makers could call employees and schedule meetings during which written proposals would be discussed. Meetings were scheduled only with proposals that the decision makers felt had problems in such areas as conceptualization, staffing, or predicted outcomes. I rarely was called to such meetings and received modest funding for my proposals. But other employees, who in my opinion had proposals that were less well thought-out and were less imaginative, were called into meetings. Further, these people received more funding than I did. I remember asking myself, "What is going on?"

After talking with many people, studying power for three years, and writing a book (Brislin, 1991), I finally figured things out. If people were called into meetings, they could argue for their proposals in a socially skilled manner and would develop positive relations with decision makers (Feeney, 2006). As a result of meetings with a positive tone, the decision makers would learn more about the proposals than was possible from just reading the written versions. Employees at the meetings could lobby for their proposals, indicating how support would benefit the decision makers. In the language of Chapter 3, the decision makers had time to develop more positive cognitions and more elaborate knowledge about the proposals at these meetings (Forgas, 2008; Hodgkinson & Healey, 2008). With these positive impressions and greater knowledge, decision makers became more familiar with the proposals and the employees who were called into the meetings. This familiarity led to more funding than those proposals that were decided based solely on their written versions.

If I had known this at the time, I would have requested a face-to-face meeting or would have taken the decision makers out to lunch. But years ago I was not as sophisticated about power and its role in decision making and so I had to work with funding less generous than some of my colleagues.

TYPES OF POWER AND POSITIVE AND NEGATIVE ASPECTS

The key to power is that it allows people to influence the behavior of others. Power can be seen in many interactions among people in the same workplace. Production line supervisors may want more attention to quality control instead of a previous emphasis on quantity alone. They have power if their wishes are followed and if the company increases its commitment to quality control. Bank managers may want to increase the number of credit cards issued to customers. They are successful with their use of power if tellers persuade large numbers of depositors to accept the bank's offer of credit cards.

Power can reside in company positions or in the people who wield power (French & Raven, 1959). There are three types of position power: legitimate, coercive, and reward. With *legitimate* power, certain individuals are recognized as having the right to direct the behavior of others. Bank managers can turn down applicants for loans. Policemen can approach an unruly crowd and ask its members to "break it up." City mayors can set priorities, such as spending money on filling potholes rather than sponsoring weekend community events at various beaches.

With *coercive* power, certain individuals can force others to behave in certain ways and have the right to administer punishment. A company's managers can fire new hires any time during an agreed-on probationary period. Coaches can bench players who break team rules. Internal Revenue Service agents can fine people who do not file their tax returns in a timely manner.

With *reward* power, certain individuals can distribute resources that people desire. Company managers can offer pay raises and promotions to employees who meet desired performance standards. College professors can award high grades to students who turn in insightful and well-written term papers. Policemen can give commendations to citizens who help in the fight against crime.

There are two types of power associated with people rather than the positions that they hold: expert and referent (French & Raven, 1959). With *expert* power, people influence others because of the knowledge and skills that they possess. Such people earn the respect of others. Office workers who know advanced computer technology that allows many employees to do their work more effectively have expert power. Pharmacists who know about interactions among various prescription drugs, and who can alert physicians to the dangers of certain drug combinations, also have this type of power.

Some people are influential because they have *referent* power. This type of power is based on people's personality and on various types of personal attractiveness. People with referent power are often exciting, interesting people who are willing to share their resources with others. In thinking about people with referent power, others make conclusions about qualities that make them good leaders—such thoughts as, "These people are very charismatic" (House et al., 2004; Yukl, 2010, and as discussed in Chapter 2). They have clear visions about a better company and they communicate their ideas clearly. They are very persuasive when they talk about what they would like to see in the future. They behave in ways that I think leaders should act. They represent the sort of person I want to be if I ever enter the ranks of leaders and powerholders.

Problems can arise when people in leadership positions are unclear about the sources of their power. For example, their status may be position-based and they may be seen as having legitimate power given their job title. But if they feel that others are deferring to them because of their personalities and other features of referent power, they may develop inflated views of themselves. Such a mistake is a major reason why some people become intoxicated and begin to abuse the power associated with their company positions (Lammers & Stapel, 2009).

The positive side of power is that leaders can use their influence to serve others and to offer improvements to their companies, communities, and churches (House et al., 2004; Yukl, 2010). The negative side of power is that it can be intoxicating and people can abuse their status. Especially when people acquire power quickly, they often have a number of predictable reactions that can cause problems. Powerful people sometimes feel that they are better than others. These powerful people become so confident in themselves that they don't ask for the suggestions of coworkers and subordinates. They take credit for the work of subordinates and do not offer public praise to hardworking employees. They sometimes think that this credit taking is justified because of their inflated view that they created the conditions that allowed subordinates to thrive. Powerful people sometimes make the mistake of derogating the work of subordinates and do not give them constructive suggestions about how to improve their work (Kipnis, 2006).

People can fall prey to these abuses of their status if they do not think carefully about the reasons for their power. People may have power because of their positions and titles, but they may erroneously feel that they have power because of their personal qualities. Powerful people often receive deference from others. Drivers slow down when they see police cars. Employees appear to listen more carefully when their bosses are talking than when coworkers are making suggestions. The drivers and employees do not always think that the policemen and bosses deserve their power because of their personal qualities. Rather, they are deferent because they feel that the policemen and bosses have legitimacy because of their positions. Some people, however, attribute the deference they receive to themselves, not their positions. They feel that they are receiving respect because of their desirable personal qualities, not their titles. Such people become especially intoxicated with power and make nuisances out of themselves (Kipnis, 2006).

How can the negative effects of power be lessened? Much like dealing with any negative behaviors that become habitual, people must want to change. They must target their negative behaviors and must avoid performing them (Baumeister & Vohs, 2007). Overweight people know that they must push themselves away from the dinner table before dessert to avoid more calories than their diets allow. Similarly, high-status people must know about the negative aspects of power and must push themselves away from temptations to abuse their positions.

THE PEOPLE WHO BECOME POWERHOLDERS

People interested in power, although often tempted to abuse it, are not necessarily evil people. In fact, they can have positive goals such as encouraging more attention to customer service in an organization or encouraging employees to become involved in community activities (House et al., 2004; Littrell, 2007). Positive aspects of power can be seen in this critical incident.

Powerful People Can Guide Others in an Ethical Manner

When people talked about George Fulton, they always had positive things to say that contributed to his reputation as "a nice guy." People in his neighborhood said that he was a pillar of the church, always ready to advise the pastor on projects that would motivate parishioners to become involved. He coached teams in the local youth basketball league, even after his own children graduated from high school. "The league was a total mess about 10 years ago," one person remembered. "George brought people together and encouraged them to put their differences aside so that the neighborhood children would have good experiences." Classmates from high school remembered George as someone who was active in student organizations. He ran for student body president and lost only because the winning candidate was an especially popular football player on a championship team.

George worked as an insurance salesman and was quite successful. He clearly cared about the well-being of his clients, and this led to many positive word-of-mouth referrals. After 12 years at his company, George was offered an executive position. He would be in charge of hiring and training new salespeople, supervising their work, and reassigning them if they did not meet their sales quotas. He would also field complaints from clients if the salespeople misrepresented the types of coverage they were offering or if they did not provide follow-up services. Occasionally, when client complaints multiplied, he would have to ask some employees to find work at another organization. Old friends wondered if George would be able to prosper in such a job given that he had such a positive reputation as a "people person."

When individuals who know George are concerned about his new position, they may have a negative view of power and wonder if a "nice guy" will find satisfaction in an administrative job. Power is not always negative. It is not a "four-letter word," so disapproved by parents that they wash their children's mouths with soap when "power" is uttered (Brislin, 1991; 2001). Power involves influencing the behavior of others. This influence can be positive or negative. Power is much like fire. Some use fire to cook their food, to heat their homes, and to provide energy for labor-saving machines. But others use it to destroy life and property. Just like power, fire is a tool that can be used for good and evil purposes (Kipnis, 2006).

Even though it may be relatively invisible, George has shown an interest in influencing others (McClelland, 1976; Winter, 1973). He enjoys advising his church's pastor. He reorganized the community basketball league, clearly having an influence on children, coaches, and parents. In high school, he campaigned for the position of student body president. This interest in working with others can be put to good use in his workplace. In his current job, George has the potential to influence many salespeople and to guide them in developing ethical business practices.

Power: The Downside. The downside of power is that its use can be intoxicating and people can become abusive in their interpersonal relationships (Brislin, 1991; Kipnis, 2006). When people drink too much alcohol, they become intoxicated and engage in behaviors that they would avoid when sober. The effects of power are similar. Many people change from friendly and decent coworkers into lunatics who find great pleasure in abusing others. This is captured in the comments people make after someone has been promoted to a company's managerial ranks. If the new manager begins to order people around, someone will surely say, "Give people a little power and it will go straight to their heads!"

David Kipnis (1976; 2006) has conducted research on other impacts of acquiring power. He found that many people find power pleasurable and strive to acquire more. People begin to make poor decisions because their judgments are clouded by their preoccupation with acquiring more influence and control over others. Powerful people begin to use company resources for their self-benefit, feeling that they are justified because they have brought so much to their organizations. These misuses of power often attract negative attention and are the first steps in people's downfalls. Newspapers often report stories of how powerholders forced employees to do work far beyond their job descriptions. Employees are asked to remodel houses, to do an executive's personal shopping, or to support a powerholder's favorite political candidate with door-to-door canvassing activities.

Powerholders either do not receive or choose to ignore negative feedback from subordinates. Consequently, they continue to behave in ways that are consistent with their inflated views of themselves. Powerholders also take too much credit for the accomplishments of subordinates. Even if they clearly do not contribute to certain successful projects, they argue that "I created the conditions under which my subordinates could prosper."

Are there steps that can be taken to lessen these negative effects of power? Yes, and one way is to establish different sets of checks and balances (Crick, 1982). If power is distributed among many people, they can enforce limits on each other. Historically, this was a reason for the rise of unions. When management abused its power, workers united to form their own influential bloc. Another way is to encourage executives to identify people who are likely to be responsible with their power. Then, they can be gradually brought into the ranks of power-holders by slowly but surely giving them more responsibilities over a number of years. When people are gradually given more power over a long period of time, sometimes called "brought along slowly," they often learn to handle its potentially intoxicating effects (Yukl, 2010).

Power as a Human Motive. When confronted with people who act in ways that are different from everyday expectations, we often ask the question, "Why did that person engage in that behavior?" With this question, we are showing an interest in people's motives. The quest for power can be a motive, and it is stronger in some people than in others (McClelland, 1976; Winter, 1973).

People's motives move them toward desired goals. Given their motives, people want to move toward goals to increase pleasure and satisfaction (McClelland, 1985). People with an affiliation motive want to be with others. They look forward to social engagements and are unhappy when they find themselves alone too often. People with an achievement motive want to complete tasks within their areas of expertise. Physicians want to perform successful operations; architects want to create award-winning designs; and writers want to have their books published. People with a nurturance motive want to help and to assist others. They often pursue careers in fields such as social work and public school teaching.

People with a power motive want to influence the behavior of others. If they make a decision, they want to see that others accept it and change their behavior so that the decision is put into practice. Power is not inherently an evil motive. Society needs people who can successfully wield power so that the public good is served. Policemen need to have their orders obeyed when they tell an unruly and aggressive group of teenagers to "break it up." If a restaurant has a reputation for serving unpalatable food by uncaring waiters, executives need their managers to follow through on directives to improve customer service. If investment companies are cheating their clients, there must be powerful people who can intervene so that investor confidence is restored (Brislin, 1991).

Power can certainly be misused. Lord Acton was correct when he warned that power can corrupt and that absolute power can corrupt absolutely (Bowman & West, 2007). Society needs various checks and balances so that no one person or collection of people can run rampant with power. For many people, the application of power creates a surge of pleasure in their brains, and so they seek out multiple opportunities to use power. These surges can become addictive, just as the pleasures brought on by drug or alcohol use can become addictive. Recognizing the dangers of power, successful executives often identify future leaders when they are in their twenties and thirties. Then, the executives assign these young people to positions with limited power. If they perform well, they are given more and more responsibility and authority in their subsequent promotions. In this way, the future leaders are "brought up slowly" to assist them in handling the temptations that accompany increasing amounts of power.

Abuses of power are not confined to headline-making events such as the Enron and WorldCom scandals. They can occur in everyday decision making. People have complained to me recently about hiring decisions. Executives chose managers without consulting with the people who would be working on a day-to-day basis with the new hire. The workers were justifiably upset. The executives may have experienced a pleasurable surge when making their decisions, but they will be hurt in the long run if they do not have the backing of employees (Watson & Michaelsen, 1984).

Impulse Control. The importance of power in the lives of some people is best understood if other motives are considered and compared with people's need for power. People with a power motive enjoy controlling the behavior of others (Winter, 1973). When powerholders make a decision, they want to see that people behave in ways consistent with their directives. In contrast, affiliative people want to socialize with others and to enjoy their company (McClelland, 1985). They look forward to interacting with others in a friendly and cordial manner. They want to be liked by others, and they often refer to themselves as "people persons."

Individuals with an achievement motive want to set and acquire goals that involve their personal efforts. Examples are students who want to receive good grades, surgeons who want to perform difficult operations, inventors who want to secure patents, and writers who want to publish books. Achievement-oriented people want to engage in activities over which they have control. They do not gamble on games where outcomes are directed by chance alone since they cannot apply their skills and lessons learned from past experiences (McClelland, 1985).

Any of these motives are well served if people can integrate impulse control. If people want to behave in certain ways but recognize they should not, then they are showing evidence of impulse control (Liddle et al., 2009). Achievement-oriented people need to nurture hobbies and to spend time with their families or else they may become burnt-out workaholics. Affiliative people often need to turn down social obligations so that they can deliver on their promises to complete work tasks by an agreed-on date. People with a power motive often need to downplay their desire to impose themselves on others. They may want to scream at their secretaries because of a costly mistake, but they realize this will be counterproductive in the long run. If bosses generate ill will and lose the support of others, they will find themselves without power. People are willing to be directed by powerholders they respect and trust, but if would-be leaders lose employee support they will become totally ineffective.

Successful leaders in large organizations have a desirable combination of the motives together with impulse control (McClelland, 1985). Their power need is high. They must find job satisfaction in directing the behavior of others. Their achievement motive cannot be so high that they become frustrated when they personally do not acquire goals through their own efforts. The job of leaders in large organizations is not to personally undertake all tasks related to company success. Their job is to make sure that others accomplish these tasks. Powerholders cannot have an affiliation motive so high that they become uncomfortable when making decisions that impact employees. For many decisions, some employees will approve and some will disapprove. Leaders have to realize that everyone cannot like them, and this can be frustrating to people with a high affiliation motive. People with impulse control (Liddle et al., 2009) can downplay the unwise and ill-considered use of power. They can recognize the intoxicating possibilities of power and can take steps to minimize them.

STRATEGIES IN THE SUCCESSFUL USE OF POWER

Once they decide that they want to enter the ranks of leaders and powerholders, people are wise to adopt some strategies for power acquisition. Strategies refer to long-range plans that involve actions in which people engage over a number of years. Four will be discussed in subsequent sections: nurturing the image of being a "winner," attending to people's faulty memories, engaging in resource acquisition for the purposes of exchanging favors, and maintaining good interpersonal relationships.

Small Wins and the Image of a "Winner." Everyone loves a winner (Weick, 1984). Aunts and uncles are much more likely to accompany parents to games if a child is playing on a winning rather than a losing soccer team. Political candidates who lose often disappear from news-paper coverage in contrast to the electoral victors. People who return home from Las Vegas after winning $50,000 receive a lot more atten-tion from friends and acquaintances than do people who lost money. The appreciation of winners also applies in the workplace.

Success through a Series of Small Wins

After graduating from Stanford with a degree in computer science, Ann Nelson interviewed at various high-tech companies in Silicon Valley and accepted a job at a software development company. A col-league told her, "I like it here because employees are encouraged to exercise their creativity and to work on self-selected projects. For exam-ple, you can work on an independent project, or you can contribute to an ongoing team effort. It'll be up to you."

If Ann accepts the career development strategy known as "small wins," she would choose to join a team effort and to make a contribu-tion to an ongoing project (Weick, 1984). The reason is that people love a winner, and small wins are enough to contribute to this reputation. If she makes a solid contribution to an ongoing team effort, she has a greater chance of being a winner than if she starts her own independ-ent project from scratch.

The fact that people love a winner can be seen in many activities. Readers might visit a youth sports program in basketball, baseball, or soccer about three-quarters of the way through a season. If a game is well attended, with many adults on both sides cheering on the young-sters, then the game will involve two teams with winning records. With winning teams, parents attend along with aunts, uncles, and family friends. But if there are only a few bedraggled-looking adults trying to appear enthusiastic, then the two teams will have losing records. Winning leads to enthusiasm and support in youth sports just as it does in people's career development.

If Ann takes on her own project during her first months at the com-pany, there is a high risk that she will not be successful and may be branded as "a loser." But if she makes a solid contribution to an ongoing project, she is far more likely to be successful. In addition, she will be able to amass various resources that she can use in the future. Working with others allows her to learn about her colleagues' skills. She will have done favors for others which may be returned in the future. She will have had time to learn the company's organizational culture (Zheng, Qu, & Yang, 2009) and to learn about the types of proj-ects that receive the most support from administrators. Too often, am-bitious people "bite off more than they can chew" during the early years of their career development. If they are less successful than they hope, they may develop a negative view of themselves. With small wins, they are more likely to make steady progress toward a successful career. With small but steady wins, they will develop a positive image among their colleagues (Weick, 1984). As a result, colleagues will offer their assistance because "everyone loves a winner."

Working with People's Faulty Memories. People may develop the image that they are winners and that they can yield power, but they have to be sure that others remember these facts. People have limited memories (Kassam, Gilbert, Swencionis, & Wilson, 2009) and power-holders are aware of this fact.

Who Are Correct? Mothers or Politicians?

The president of the financial services company where Carol Summers worked asked her to orient a new employee. Carol scheduled a meeting with Steve Burris during his second day at work. When talking about the company and the experiences of employees, Carol found that she was drawing from her memories of what happened during her first six months at the company. Or, she found that she talked about what had been happening during the last three weeks. Since she had worked at the company for eight years, Carol wondered if she was overemphasizing events that occurred early and very recently in her employment.

Carol has encountered issues related to primacy and recency (Duffy & Crawford, 2008). When people enter life experiences that are unfamiliar, they remember what happened very early during these experiences. This is called the *primacy effect*. For example, people remember events during the first few months of a new job. During these months, they want to learn company norms and the rules for being considered a success. Since they learn these critical issues during their early months, events that led to the learning stick in their minds. After they learn company norms and rules, they no longer need to have detailed memories of their day-to-day experiences in their company.

In addition to good memories for early experiences, people remember what happened to them recently. People can tell what they had for dinner two nights ago, but probably not on a specific date two months ago. Recent events are still fresh in people's minds and people can tell others about them. In addition to her early experiences in the company, Carol can tell Steve about interesting events that have occurred during the last few weeks. This is called the *recency effect*.

Primacy and recency can be seen in the advice given by mothers and politicians. Mothers tell their children, "Behave well when you meet people for the first time since first impressions are lasting." Mothers are correct because they are giving advice based on primacy. Early encounters with unfamiliar others will stick in people's minds. People want to come to conclusions about individuals they have just met. Since there is no long background of encounters, early events have a great impact.

Seasoned politicians tell less-experienced colleagues, "Be ready to tell voters what you have done for them during the six months prior to your reelection. Don't expect them to remember what you did two years ago." These politicians are also correct and are basing their advice on the recency effect (Duffy & Crawford, 2008). People have many experiences listening to politicians and know what impresses them and what does not. Given that they have to vote for many candidates running for different offices, people cannot be expected to remember everything about the candidates. Voters are likely to remember what has happened recently when they make choices among a slate of candidates.

Resources and Resource Acquisition. People with power are able to compete for scarce resources in their workplaces, communities, and political organizations. Whenever people want scarce resources, they must enter political arenas (Smith, 1988). Such arenas are not limited to the activities of Democrats, Republicans, and smaller groups that want to have an impact on legislation and public policy. When people talk about "office politics" (Drory & Romm, 1990) or "political goings-on in this voluntary organization," they are talking about the competition for resources. People who possess knowledge of how power works have an advantage in this competition.

There are various types of resources that people use as "currency," and they must possess one or more to be taken seriously by power-holders. I'll use the example of people seeking political office, but applications can be made to other arenas such as a workplace where consumers find goods or services. The clearest scarce resource is money. There are only so many jobs that pay salaries of $100,000 or more. There is only so much money that people are willing to donate to political campaigns. Another resource is services. Elected politicians are expected to serve the needs of people in their districts. The relation between money and services provides a good introduction to a key aspect of the political process. People with power trade resources (Foa, 1971; Roussseau, 2001). Politicians ask for money for their campaigns. Those donating money expect that the politicians will work hard for members of the electorate. Whether or not politicians give more services and large government contracts to generous campaign donors is an endlessly debated topic among activists, journalists, and politicians themselves.

Another resource is goods. People with access to food and sound equipment at wholesale costs will have access to politicians who want to stage community events. Information is an important resource. Before these events, politicians often ask local leaders about issues of current concern among a community's voters. The politicians integrate this information into their speeches at the public events. Without this key information, the politicians would come across as "out of touch" with the voters in any one specific community.

People who want to enter powerful circles for the first time must think through the resources that they can offer (Foa, 1971). Again, the clearest example is money. People who have money and show a willingness to donate to political campaigns will be invited to fund-raisers and will find themselves seated among the community's movers and shakers. If they are all clever, they will participate in discussions about government land deals and various investment opportunities and will be able to increase their wealth. For people who do not see large amounts of money in their futures, information is the best resource to develop and to offer. Elected politicians cannot possess detailed information about all issues that need government attention. They need to surround themselves with people who have expertise about such issues as drug policy, public school education, and economic development. People who develop an expertise in these issues, and who are able to communicate it clearly, can trade their knowledge for access to power-holders (Smith, 1988).

Good Interpersonal Relationships. Although it certainly can have a dark side, the use of power does not always have negative connotations. Many tactics of powerholders are ethical, make good common sense, and should be learned by all workers. These include clear communication of one's ideas (Chapters 4 and 5), the development of positive relations with others in the workplace (Thomas & Inkson, 2009), the willingness to help others with their proposals, and the knowledge that one should be careful about returning favors (Rousseau, 2001). Assume that a person has an innovative proposal for new directions that an organization could pursue. If the person presents the proposal clearly, and has the support from others based on good interpersonal relations, then the proposal is likely to receive careful consideration.

Mistakes in Interpersonal Exchanges

With this background, let's consider a short example. Dan Bennett was the influential president of a technology firm in San Francisco. Given his extensive volunteer efforts, he was well known in many influential circles. Jane Freeman recently graduated from a college in

Illinois. She had played on a high-school volleyball team with Dan's daughter. On returning to San Francisco, Jane called Dan and asked him for an appointment. She wanted to discus job possibilities and asked Dan for a letter of recommendation. Dan agreed, wrote the letter, and Jane soon landed a job. Dan heard about Jane's job because his daughter mentioned it one night at dinner. About 18 months later, Jane called Dan again, this time asking that he sponsor her for membership in a local organization of business professionals. Dan was uncomfortable with this request.

Jane has made several mistakes in her search for a career in her community. She has not kept up communication with Dan (Chapters 5 and 6). She did not seek out ways of returning the favor Dan gave her when he wrote the letter of recommendation (Foa, 1971; Rousseau, 2001). After an 18-month period of silence, sometimes called a "disappearing act," Dan is understandably upset when Jane requests a second favor. He may think to himself, "If she is careless with me about keeping up communication and maintaining professional relations, she may behave in these ways toward other influential people in the community."

When people work toward important goals in the workplace and in their communities, they almost always need to involve others. People who have developed positive interpersonal relations have an advantage in the pursuit of their goals (Borman, 2004; Watson & Michaelsen, 1984). These relationships should be carefully nurtured. Benjamin Franklin wrote that people who do not socialize with others when they go to a tavern may find themselves alone when they need help to find their horses. A similar sentiment applies to today's boardrooms. People who have not developed positive relations with coworkers may experience silence when they offer their proposals at meetings of company executives.

TACTICS IN THE USE OF POWER

Tactics refer to carefully inserted behaviors that are part of a person's desire to use power. Whereas strategies refer to long-range plans, the use of any one tactic is usually shorter in duration and is chosen because of its usefulness at a given time and in a specific place. Some tactics are dark and manipulative and I do not recommend their use (Brislin, 1991). However, I recommend that people know about manipulative tactics so that they can recognize them when they are the targets of ethically challenged power seekers.

Agenda Setting. Readers might examine their memories and consider whether or not this tactic has been used against them. In my own quest to understand power, I now recognize that I have been a victim of "agenda setting" several times in the distant past.

Unknown Power Tactics Place Employees at a Disadvantage

Janet Moore, the president of a brokerage firm, established a policy of inviting one mid-level employee to each monthly meeting of the company's vice presidents. For the next meeting Kathy Tanabe was invited, and Janet asked her to talk to colleagues about issues that they would like to see covered. Kathy did so, and prepared a proposal for improvements in the company's medical care coverage benefits. Even though Janet preferred not discussing this issue, she agreed to put it on the meeting's agenda.

Janet scheduled the meeting for 11:00 A.M. on a Friday. She placed Kathy's proposal as the seventh topic to be discussed. Other items, higher on the agenda, included salaries, sharing of commissions when two people were involved in a sale, parking privileges, and policies regarding sexual harassment in the workplace. The meeting continued until 12:30 P.M., and the senior people decided to break for lunch. While disappointed that her proposal was not covered during the meeting, Kathy was pleased that it had been scheduled for discussion.

Kathy has been the victim of a tactic called "agenda setting" (Brislin, 1991). Janet does not want to discuss the issue of medical care coverage, but she does not want to be seen as unresponsive to her employees' proposals. So she schedules the meeting at 11:00 A.M. and places a number of time-consuming items early on the agenda. From her experience, Janet knows that items such as the sharing of commissions and sexual harassment will generate extensive discussions. She also knows that by 12:30 P.M. people's hunger pangs will lead to a request for an end to the meeting so that they can go to lunch. Janet reaps two benefits. Employees see her as willing to listen to their concerns, and she is able to continue ignoring the issue of medical benefits.

This is the sort of tactic that "goes right over people's heads" unless they have a very sophisticated understanding of power in the workplace. I have seen this tactic used many times, and employees rarely see that executives implement it to ignore issues that they do want to have discussed. Although there are no guaranteed ways to counter this tactic, the following scenario will sometimes work. Kathy schedules a short meeting with Janet the next week. Very politely, she says, "Thank you very much for scheduling the medical benefits proposal on the agenda. It's too bad that we didn't have enough time at the meeting to cover it. I hope that you can put it higher on the agenda at next month's meeting." By making this suggestion, Kathy is showing that she knows about the agenda setting tactic, but at the same time she is being polite and showing respect for Janet's position. Possibly, Janet will recognize Kathy as being knowledgeable about power and will not use this tactic a second time. Kathy may also improve her position in the company. The combination of "polite, respectful, and sophisticated about power" is highly valued in organizations. Kathy can show that she should be placed on the fast track for promotion if she deals with power tactics in a way that demonstrates her awareness and social skills.

Machiavellian Tactics. Some tactics for the acquisition and maintenance of power were identified by Niccolo Machiavelli in his classic book, *The Prince* (reprinted, 1940).

Machiavellian Tactics Are Too Often Seen in the Workplace

Wanting changes made in the organization he owned, Martin Snyder knew that he would be unpopular if he was seen as the major agent of his plans for the future. The changes involved a reorganization of the company, layoffs, modifications of employees' job descriptions, and transfers to a branch office 30 miles from some employees' homes. So Martin hired John Fletcher and gave him the title of vice president for administration. John talked to all the employees and seemed attentive and concerned about people's welfare. After a month, John instituted the exact changes that Martin had in mind all along. Employees began to complain, but Martin told them, "To be fair to John, we have to give him some time to see if his changes bring improvements to the company."

After a year, the organization's remaining employees called a meeting with Martin to update their complaints. Martin listened carefully, then agreed to fire John. Employees were extremely pleased and felt that Martin had made a tough decision with their best interests in mind. However, by the time Martin fired John all of his desired changes were in place. Employees had become tolerant of the changes and agreed that it would be even more upsetting and confusing to go back to the old ways. Martin reaped multiple benefits. His changes were in place but he was not seen as the major source of unpopular company policies. He became a hero in the eyes of his employees for firing John, who had earned the title of "this organization's hatchet man."

This tactic was described by Niccolo Machiavelli in his classic book, *The Prince*. Machiavelli was born in Florence and lived during the late 15th and early 16th centuries. He was a civil servant who held a variety of posts, and he was a very astute observer of human behavior. By writing observations about how a ruler could acquire and maintain power, he felt that he would gain favor from members of the influential Medici family. At the time of Machiavelli's observations concerning power, Florence was politically unstable and there were constant threats from various usurpers who wanted to dispose of any current ruler. Machiavelli gave advice that he thought was practical in the context of this instability. People who ignore the times in which he lived accuse Machiavelli of power strategies that favor manipulation and treachery over ethics, decency, and respect for people being governed (Christie & Geis, 1970; Dahling, Whitaker, & Levy, 2009). For this reason, manipulative and backstabbing tactics in the workplace have become known as "Machiavellian."

This tactic involving the behaviors of Martin Snyder and John Fletcher is not one that I would recommend. Over the long run, given today's world where good employees can leave an organization and find work elsewhere, such tactics can work against an employer's goals. Executives who use such tactics will develop a negative reputation and will not be able to attract good employees. Executives may be able to use such schemes once or twice, but will damage themselves if use of the tactics becomes habitual. This is especially true in small communities where people know each other, talk about each other, and have very good memories for abusive behaviors that were directed at them.

Appealing to Unseen High-Level Decision Makers. In the previous incident, Martin passed the dirty work of organizational layoffs to John. Powerholders often manipulate interactions with subordinates to come across as "the good guy" while directing employee animosity at an unseen and unavailable target.

Appeals to Boogeymen Can Derail Controversial Proposals

As part of the yearly budgeting process, senior staff members of a social services agency met to develop plans for the upcoming year. They also discussed projects that were successful over the last year and tried to diagnose the reasons for projects where expectations were not met. After this meeting, plans would be shared with the agency's executive board, which was composed of well-known businesspeople and other influential community members. The agency's director, Rose Watanabe, asked her staff for suggestions. One of the younger social workers on staff, Ann Deever, suggested that resources be allocated to the development of homeless villages for people currently living on the streets.

Rose did not want to consider this proposal, but she listened carefully to Ann's arguments. Privately, Rose felt that the proposal would generate too much political opposition from taxpayers who lived in areas near homeless villages. Rose had experienced the NIMBY problem in the past. People want to help the poor and the homeless, but "not in my backyard." But Ann pressed on with her proposal, citing successes in other states where similar projects had been introduced. Rose wanted to encourage Ann, a good employee, but at the same time did not want to pursue the homeless village issue. So Rose said, "Ann, I am all in favor of your proposal. But I don't think the executive board will approve it. They are not ready for a proposal like this. Maybe, as public opinion changes, they will be more sympathetic in the future."

Rose is using a tactic known as bringing in the boogeyman (Brislin, 1991). This character, who made an appearance in the Laurel and Hardy version of *Babes in Toyland,* is a creature who parents have reportedly used to discipline children. "If you don't eat your spinach, or do your homework, the boogeyman will come and get you." Since this character is rarely seen except on the late-late show after children have gone to bed, it remains a rather vague but threatening punishment in children's minds. This vagueness remains when boogeymen are employed in today's organizations. Rose might not have the slightest idea about the feelings of the executive board concerning a proposal for homeless villages. But she can discourage Ann from pursuing her ideas by appealing to the negative reactions of influential people. Rose benefits in several ways. She is seen as supporting Ann by saying that she is personally in favor of the proposal. In addition, she avoids further discussion of an issue that she wants to see tabled for the indefinite future.

Appealing to a boogeyman is a tactic that can sometimes be countered. If she knows of its existence, Ann can approach Rose. She can say, "I appreciate your support of the proposal, and it's too bad about the executive board. Can you give me contact information for some of the board members so that I can talk to them personally and possibly deal with their concerns?" By responding in this manner, Ann is communicating that she knows about the tactic but is not challenging Rose's authority directly. Possibly, Rose will recognize Ann's sophistication and will not use such tactics in the future.

Passing the Buck Concerning Decisions That May Be Unpopular.
Tactics that powerholders use to make themselves look good and a subordinate look bad (Lambert, 2008) are so common that they deserve further discussion.

Making Someone Else the Bad Guy Has Developed into an Art Form

"It's time we made some changes that may be unpopular with some of the employees," Herb Jenkins told Julie Benson. Herb was the president and chief executive officer of a company that both manufactured and sold clothing for men, women, and children. Julie was his vice president for administration. Herb knew that some of his proposed changes would affect the jobs of some people and could lead to layoffs. He asked Julie to develop a staffing plan based on his ideas for changes. After two months, Julie presented the plan to Herb. Both agreed that three people had to be told that their services would no longer be required.

Julie talked to the three people individually and gave them the bad news. Two of the employees had already decided to leave the company because of family commitments in other states. The third pink-slipped employee made an appointment with Herb and pleaded his case. He pointed out that there were limited opportunities for jobs in his specialized field of information technology, and that he would have to leave the state to find comparable employment. He continued that his two children were in high school and that he did not want to make them leave their friends and transfer to another school. Herb relented and agreed to retain the information technology specialist. Word got around the organization that Julie was the mean-spirited demon who wanted to fire people and that Herb saved the day with his intervention.

Herb has shown that he is the master of an art form. Even though both Herb and Julie agreed that the personnel changes were necessary, one of the two people emerged from the exercise with a positive reputation in the company (Machiavelli, 1940). I have seen this technique used a number of times. An administrator wants changes, asks an assistant to put the changes into practice, and then relents when there is rebellion. The person who communicated to employees that they should seek employment elsewhere is left "holding the bag" and becomes known as a "hatchet man" (whether the person is male or female).

Employers often do not want to be seen as the origin of decisions that impact employees in a negative manner. So, consciously or unconsciously, they give this task to someone else who then becomes the target of resentment. What are the benefits of this process for Julie and other vice presidents? Why don't they quit their jobs in disgust? For some, they feel that they are well paid and that they could not do better financially if they put themselves on the job market. For others, they view communicating negative decisions as part of their preparation for a higher position. For still others, they view this distasteful task as showing their loyalty to the company president. Many "number two people" feel that they will be the chosen successor when the current president retires or moves on. When I counsel vice presidents who are frustrated given experiences similar to Julie's, I tell them that I hope that they are 100 percent confident of their president's intentions. Presidents who manipulate their subordinates into "holding the bag" for unpopular decisions are ethically challenged. If they are willing to engage in this behavior, they may be willing to set aside promises made to a vice president concerning career development leading to the chief executive officer position.

The use of problematic tactics such as those described in the last pages of this chapter will eventually bring misery to an organization. People will not trust each other. They will not know what communications to believe and which to ignore. Middle-level managers will not know what information should be passed on to their subordinates

8

Social Skills

In the last three chapters, we have discussed the importance of good communication skills in the workplace, as well as sophisticated political skills. Working effectively with other people and gaining their respect are two outcomes of communication skills and political savvy. A related set of workplace essentials is summarized by the term *social skills* (Baron & Tang, 2009; Karnes, 2009). Many of these are only slightly advanced versions of what our parents tried to teach us as we matured through a carefree childhood, grew into angst-filled teenagers, and emerged as young adults. Don't many of us remember our parents' attempts to instill politeness, to send thank-you notes for gifts, to make good first impressions, and to learn ways of interacting smoothly with a wide variety of people? Our parents undoubtedly wanted us to learn our social skills, but this might have been a difficult task given our reticence to learn and given the many other demands on their time.

Whether fully or only partially successful, our parents were trying to prepare us for a basic fact of life. Virtually all tasks in today's workplaces require that individuals interact with many others during the course of a day (Uchitelle, 2007). These others include coworkers, customers, clients, supervisors, and members of advisory boards who have an influence on organizational policy making. The ability to work well with others is facilitated by social skills. In years past, children learned social skills at home. Parents taught children proper table manners, rules of etiquette such as thank-you letters on receiving gifts, ways of making visitors feel welcome, conversational skills for social gatherings, and so forth. As more and more parents became dual wage earners, social skills training at home became a low-priority item. Some schools picked up the slack, but social skills training had to compete with the hours necessary to master traditional school subjects. Adults who feel they missed out on their social skills can now take courses offered by profit-making companies.

When workers are promoted to managerial ranks, social skills are required (Uchitelle, 2007). I have been on many selection committees for managerial positions, and people's ability to work well with others is always discussed. When workers become managers, they do not carry out all tasks themselves. Rather, the managers make sure that the tasks are done. The managers must assign the tasks to others and provide the necessary support to subordinates. They must supervise, but not actually do the work. Social skills such as showing respect for subordinates, communicating with them about progress on the tasks, and knowing when to intervene without embarrassing subordinates become essential.

Social skills are different from intellectual skills. Consider people who are clearly smart in the sense of their formal education. They have a large vocabulary, read several newspapers daily, can do complex mathematical calculations without consulting a book, and can cite obscure literary figures during their everyday conversations. But they can't get along with coworkers in their organizations. They cannot communicate what they would like to see happen. They irritate others so much that they are avoided like the plague. These people may be book smart, but they are lacking in people skills (Sternberg, 1986; Goleman, 1997).

As people develop various skills that are useful in their lives, they become better able to attain their goals. As they develop their verbal skills, they find themselves able to learn more from their reading and to communicate better through their writing and oral presentations. As they develop their musical abilities, they find themselves invited to social gatherings where they are asked to play their instruments. As they develop their athletic skills, they find themselves feeling better because they are in good physical condition.

When individuals develop better social skills, they discover that more people are willing to interact with them and to help them on various projects at work and in their communities. Social skills allow individuals to benefit from the contributions others can make. Problems arise when people forget or neglect social skills and, as a result, irritate and possibly alienate others.

Additional social skills are necessary when managers want to pursue projects that involve widespread company change (Uchitelle, 2007). Managers can direct subordinates to accept tasks related to the new projects, but they can rarely order fellow managers to pursue new goals in the organization. When working with fellow managers, they need to persuade others rather than to direct them. This means that any one manager has to listen carefully to the thoughts of coworkers whose support is desired (Strauss, 2006). When I give training programs dealing with workplace enjoyment, many people respond to my request for descriptions about absences of social skills. Faulty listening skills (Bays, 2007) were one theme in people's anecdotes. A businessperson in Honolulu wrote, "Another manager wanted my support. We set up a meeting about a week in advance. At the appointed time, he called me from his cell phone. He said he was in his car and on his way into a parking lot. He told me he had a few minutes and asked if the telephone call could substitute for the scheduled meeting. I was so stunned that I continued the phone conversation. I had prepared some visual aids for the meeting that, of course, I could not use during the phone conversation. I felt that he blew me off with this meeting substitution. I did not become involved in his project, and have not become involved in any of his subsequent ideas."

Another businessman once told me, "Especially communities where you are likely to encounter the same people year after year, what goes around comes around. If you don't treat people well, they won't treat you well." To this astute observation, I would add that people have long memories. If the poor treatment occurred 20 years ago, people will still remember it today and make decisions about project involvement based on these memories.

SOME BASIC SOCIAL SKILLS

People can use some skills again and again rather than on only a few occasions a month. One is careful listening. I'll examine this skill in comparing good and less able managers in the workplace.

Listening to Others. When workers schedule a meeting with managers, they almost always have concerns that they want to share. Managers should listen carefully to workers (Bays, 2007), should not interrupt, and should take steps to ensure that the workers have voiced all their concerns. Managers should make sure that they are showing respect for the workers' concerns. Workers often have to dredge up all their courage before making appointments to voice their positions, and so managers should make the workers feel that everyone's time is being well spent.

This piece of advice may seem to be little more than common sense, but workers often complain that their managers do not listen carefully. If it is common sense, it is a point missed by many managers. The advice also can be at odds with a conversational style during highly informal talks with friends. As part of friendly, informal interactions, people often engage in conversational overlap. People make statements, and before they end someone else jumps in. Often, this takes the form of one person starting a sentence and someone else finishing it. This overlap can continue for many rounds, with the first person who spoke interrupting others as they add to the conversation.

This overlapping style is widely accepted and is not considered rude when it is used during informal social events. The style is meant to show that people have much in common since they can add to the same conversation. In addition, no one person becomes the center of attention since everyone is participating in the informal conversation and is contributing to an enjoyable social occasion.

The difference between the manager-worker conversation style and the overlapping style is that one is formal and the other is not. When people have a concern that they want to share with managers, they do not want to participate in the informal overlapping style. They want the full attention of managers (Bays, 2007; Hodgkinson & Healey, 2008). The informal style is more common outside the workplace. People use it interacting at company picnics, watching their children play youth sports, and at chance meetings at shopping malls.

To make matters more complex, managers should sometimes participate in the overlapping style. When they have lunch with workers or share the coffeepot with them, appropriate behavior is more informal than formal. How do managers tell the difference? This is another social skill. When workers speak with managers, they may want to talk informally or they may want to bring up a burning issue. Managers need to read nonverbal cues (Hall, 1959; 1966), such as facial expressions, relaxed compared to tense body postures, and the types of gestures people use while speaking. Like all social skills, decisions about appropriate conversational styles can be improved if people have the desire and are willing to invest the necessary time and effort.

Developing a Network. Executives from various private and nonprofit organizations frequently give presentations at nearby university business schools. These executives are often asked about advice for career development. Responses include recommendations such as "join student organizations, seek out internship possibilities, volunteer for community service activities, and become more active in organizations such as your church and political party." If people follow this advice, they will increase the size of their networks and will reap positive benefits. Some people, however, don't know what a network is and don't know how it differs from family and friends.

Networks consist of people who exchange favors with each other (Brislin, 1991; Foa, 1971). By calling on network members, people increase their chances of effectiveness in their workplace (Aparna, 2006). People in a network do not have to be close friends who spend much of their free time together. Their goal is to offer various types of help, and they can do this with only one or two contacts per year. For example, assume that a person wants to learn about local business opportunities that could form the basis for entrepreneurial ventures. If that person has a good network, she can call on various members. One network member may know the name of a journalist who has written about small businesses. Another member may know business professors at a nearby business school who advise entrepreneurs. Another may know the names of venture capitalists looking for investment opportunities. The most effective networks have members from many different backgrounds who can offer various types of information, advice, and names of others to contact. People become involved in networks through the types of activities recommended by executives: joining various organizations, internships, and working on political campaigns (Brislin, 1991; Foa, 1971).

Some people in small communities, especially if they are from large extended families, don't feel the need to network. They already have enough aunts, uncles, cousins, and old family friends to call on when help is needed. This may be true for a few fortunate individuals. Most people, however, need to move beyond their extended families if they are to meet the lawyers, professors, physicians, politicians, and businesspeople that constitute the membership of an effective network.

In addition to developing their network, people must learn about the expectations of members (Oh, Chung, & Labianca, 2004). People in the same network trade favors (Cialdini, 2001). It is enjoyable to be on the receiving end of favors, but people must learn how to offer favors when appropriate. If young professionals are fortunate enough to have senior executives in their network, how might they return favors? One way is to find out about the executives' community activities. If young professionals join and help community organizations that the executives support, they are showing their gratitude and are returning favors through their time and effort. They are also likely to increase their networks even more through the other people they will meet during voluntary efforts for the community organizations.

Showing Respect for Others. Many social skills that managers should possess involve showing respect for coworkers and subordinates (Strauss, 2006; Smith, 2008). For many people, respect is like money: they don't get as much as they would like. When the comedian Rodney Dangerfield was trying to make his mark as a major figure in show business, he tried out various types of jokes to see what worked best with audiences. He found that when he emphasized that others failed to appreciate and to pay attention to him, audiences responded with laughter. This became summarized in his trademark phrase, "I don't get no respect." One of his jokes: "I went to see the doctor and he said I was fat and had to go on a diet. I told him I wanted a second opinion. He said, 'Okay, you're ugly too!'" After one show, Jack Benny came backstage to see Rodney. The older comedian advised Rodney to emphasize the "lack of respect" material. He pointed out that all audience members can relate to this since a lack of respect is part of everyone's life at one time or another (Dangerfield, 2004)

In the workplace, managers can show respect by listening carefully to subordinates. As long as it is a sincere gesture rather than a piece of theatrical fluff, managers can take notes while the subordinates speak. Managers also need to show that they respect the employees' time and do not want to communicate that they have something more important to do. If employees schedule a meeting that they feel will last a half-hour, they are going to be irritated if managers look at their watches after about 10 minutes. If managers have to look at their watches, they must give the employees a reason. For instance, they must say that they are expecting a light knock on the door from a secretary who has a folder of materials related to the employees' concerns.

If managers make a commitment during the meeting, they must follow through on their promises. Even if they have nothing to report after about two weeks, employees appreciate a memo or e-mail saying, "I don't have anything to report as a follow-up to our meeting, but I am still working on the issues you raised. I'll get back to you again when I have more information."

Responding to Invitations. When I ask successful managers to tell me about social skills that would benefit from improvement, there is no dearth of suggestions (Cortes, 2000). One told me, "Please start with the lack of response to RSVP requests on invitations. I send out invitations for a business luncheon that my company is sponsoring. We ask invitees to tell us whether or not they will be coming. This seems like a pretty reasonable request since we have to tell the caterers how many lunches to prepare. But it ends up being guesswork. Sometimes plenty of people just show up and I don't eat lunch since I give mine to someone else."

This is a common problem in communities where people think that they know a large number of people, but in actuality this number is a small percentage of the community's total population. Most of my students are in their twenties and so marriage is possible in their not-so-distant futures. I tell them, "Ladies and gentlemen, there will be a time in a few years when you will be very frustrated. In fact, if there are guns around you might use them inappropriately. You will be planning your wedding and will send out invitations and, of course, you will want people to tell whether they are coming or not. But you won't hear from a lot of people. Consequently, in addition to the time demands of all your other wedding plan activities, you or a relative will have to get on the phone and ask if invitees are coming."

I believe that the lack of emphasis on RSVP social skills comes from people's belief that they were born and raised in a small community, but in actuality the community has grown beyond the small size etched into their memories. In addition, the number of places where people might see each other was also small in past years: the shopping center, the museum, or one of a few big movie theaters. Now, there are many shopping centers, art galleries and museums, and small suburban theaters have replaced yesterday's large downtown movie palaces. In the past, people could run into each other and say, "Oh yes, I'll come to the business lunch." Now, people are in so many different places that they are far less likely to see each other.

Problems arise because some people have not yet developed the habit of sending a note or placing a telephone call to substitute for the lack of a face-to-face meeting. Perhaps today's users of sophisticated technology will contribute to social skills improvement (Lipscomb, Totten, Cook, & Lesch, 2007). With today's cell phones, sending short RSVP text messages is simple and consumes very little time. The message that "I can come" or "Sorry, I can't come" will probably be delivered through means other than the letters and phone calls of the past.

Keeping Up Contact with Favor Givers. A frequently forgotten social skill is that people have obligations if influential individuals offer assistance on tasks such as job searches and letters of recommendation for professional awards (Cialdini, 2001). Those obligations include progress reports on the job search and activities related to the possible awards, thank-you letters no matter the outcomes, and attempts to return favors.

One high-level and successful manager told me, "I often find myself giving advice to young job seekers. They make appointments, come to my office, and I tell them what I know about the current job market. But then I rarely hear from them again. It's as if they do a disappearing act. So I don't know whether they got a job or not. After a few years, I might see them at one meeting or another. But even then they don't come over and tell me what has happened to them. Such experiences make it less likely that I will be enthusiastic about helping other job seekers in the future."

This is a common complaint. Social skills clearly call for continued contact with people who have helped in the past. I feel that one reason for the lack of continuous contact is that the job seekers, or in general favor seekers, do not want to be remembered as once needing help. If these individuals now have a job or have received an award, their current accomplishments are what they want others to have in mind. These individuals do not want to be remembered as unemployed job seekers or as people wanting favors.

The lack of follow-up contact has negative effects. People who have favors to offer become jaded and sometimes avoid professional gatherings where they might be the targets of requests for their resources. Another executive pointed out, "I sometimes dread going to business meetings where lunch will be served or where there will be a long coffee break. Some people seem to treat these meetings as places where they can hustle up favors. These people treat others like deer during open hunting season. They target influential individuals and then go after them. And of course, they never think of doing anything to return the favors they receive."

Today's communication technologies such as e-mail and text-messaging make keeping in touch very easy (Lipscomb et al., 2006). In addition to letting favor givers know about the progress made given their advice or recommendations, beneficiaries can describe their efforts to return favors. Often, influential people with favors to give are very busy and so cannot give time to all of the community organizations whose leaders request their help. Those helped by these influential people can return favors by volunteering and spending time in these organizations. There are always volunteer activities for people willing to spend time with organizations such as the Blood Bank, Meals on Wheels, and Boy and Girl Scouts. Influential people are impressed by individuals who strive to return favors, and they will remember these activities when they have other resources to share in the future (Brislin, 1991).

ADVANCED SOCIAL SKILLS

The skills discussed up to this point are not far removed from what parents try to instill in their children. There are other skills that go beyond the teachings of parents, and these might be called "advanced social skills." Many of these have to be developed outside of the home. The first skill stems from a certainty that all managers will face. No matter how hard they try to please everyone, they cannot (Beyer et al., 1997; Kinicki & Williams, 2008). This means that some of the decisions will be criticized. The advanced social skill that managers should nurture is to respond to criticism with a well-developed thick skin.

Accepting Criticism. Employees appreciate bosses who are able to encourage participation from workers and who can integrate their suggestions into better company policies (Pencavel, 2003). Workers also appreciate bosses who listen carefully and who show respect for employee contributions. With many managers, there is a potential difficulty. If bosses encourage participation, they will surely hear some suggestions with which they disagree or which imply criticism of their past management practices. Even if there is no direct confrontation, especially sensitive people may feel that they are being criticized for not thinking of the suggestion themselves. Bosses have to develop thick skins if they are to encourage participative decision making.

People with aspirations for managerial positions are well advised to engage in a self-examination regarding the thickness of their skins. Questions to pose include, "Can I accept criticism of my work? Can I disagree with people on social and political issues and retain a calm demeanor? In other words, can I disagree with people without being disagreeable? If I am in a public setting, can I be criticized by a large number of people and still keep my poise?" If answers to these and related questions is "no," people should consider engaging in activities that might thicken up their skins.

One method is to take courses in public speaking and in facilitating group discussions, and these are often offered through the outreach programs of colleges and universities. Another method is to join community organizations and to volunteer for committee work where people will surely disagree. If they volunteer for committees that deal with the finances of volunteer organizations where members pay dues, they will be able to take advantage of a quirky aspect of human behavior. Even if people are quite wealthy, they are very sensitive about how their money is spent when they pay dues to an organization. If the organization collects $50 a year from each member, the money can be spent on a yearly dinner, trip to a tourist attraction, or plants to make the downtown area of their communities more attractive. No matter what the suggestion, some member will disagree. Defending one's own suggestion and listening respectfully to the ideas presented by others provide good learning experiences for career development (Kurzman, 2009).

Developing a thick skin may be harder in small communities than in other parts of the United States (Brislin, 2008). The adage "people who live in glass houses shouldn't throw stones" sometimes leads to gentleness and softness when offering criticism of others. For example, interactions in Hawaii are often marked by a soft tone. One of the people I work with closely recently interviewed for jobs outside of Hawaii. He reported, "The questions I was asked were much tougher than anything I had experienced in Hawaii. I think I handled them O.K., but I had to draw from my experiences that I had in Oregon, before I came to Hawaii." From my observations, this is an issue frequently faced by people who have spent most of their lives in small communities. It reinforces the advice to examine one's ability to accept suggestions for improvement and to deal with criticism. If people generate self-insights that identify problem areas, they can take steps to improve.

Responding to Employee Suggestions. If managers are unable to accept criticism and to respond to employee suggestions for improvement, they may end up as characters reminiscent of a *Dilbert* comic strip. The theme behind many frustrations in *Dilbert* is that managers often ask for worker opinions but actually don't want to hear anything but their own voices.

One of my colleagues remembers a boss he had in an organization where he once worked. This manager would stroll up to a worker's desk, knock his knuckles on the cubicle wall, and would ask, "How are you doing?" At this point, it did not make any difference what the worker said. The manager would go directly into his predetermined topic of conversation. He would very slowly draw out a single point that he wanted to get across, taking 20 minutes to do so. A more efficient person would cover the same material in five minutes. My colleague continued, "There were never conversations because it was a one-way flow of information. No matter what you said during the conversation, he would just plow ahead with his point. He seemed to have little regard for people's feedback or expertise, and he was unable to show respect for people's time." The employees would share ideas among themselves concerning how best to deal with these unhelpful meetings. They decided that the most efficient action would be to say nothing and to hope that the meetings would end as soon as possible.

Another colleague described the behavior of his boss at departmental meetings. The boss would ask employees to prepare reports on various company activities. After he opened the meeting and gave his own reports, he would sit back and engage in activities other than listening carefully to the employees. For instance, he would cut his fingernails when others were presenting their carefully prepared reports.

I have tremendous empathy for these people since I once had the misfortune of working for a boss who likewise showed little interest in the contributions of employees. She would call meetings and present her own ideas. Then, she would spend the rest of the allotted meeting time trying to force a jolly and cheerful mood. Employees who had serious issues to raise had to endure this false gaiety. If they were successful in their attempts to cover serious issues, they came across as Ebenezer Scrooge-like characters who couldn't enjoy a convivial meeting.

This person later ran for public office and was criticized by the media for her poor performance in handling the rough and tumble that is an inevitable part of political campaigning. I believe that if she had been responsive to her employees in her earlier job, she would have benefited from practice in showing respect to others (Kurzman, 2009), handling difficult questions, and remaining calm when challenged (Brislin, 1991).

If managers want to be known as both effective and cooperative in the workplace, they must listen carefully when employees have concerns (Bays, 2007). They must tell employees which concerns they will be able to address and then follow through on their commitments. Further, they should heed the advice that is central to the stories in this section concerning workplace social skills. "If you don't want to hear employee suggestions, don't go through the facade of asking for them."

Working a Crowd. I would now like to turn to an advanced social skill that I do not possess. This is the ability to go to social events where individuals want to interact with others but know few people in attendance. Despite the fact that individuals have not previously met others at the gathering, they can interact smoothly with multiple attendees and have a good time. This talent is sometimes called the ability to "work a crowd." This is a skill that is possessed by relatively few people, but it is worth discussing since those who possess it have an edge in the quest for executive-level positions. To start the discussion, I need to return to a topic introduced earlier in this chapter: The importance of networks.

People often reap great benefits if they have good networks in their communities (Aparna, 2006; Cohen & Janicki-Deverts, 2009; Foa, 1971). If people know many other individuals, they have access to knowledge that may not be generally known. They also may have access to favors that influential individuals can grant. In addition, these influential community leaders can "talk up" favored people and can contribute to their positive reputations. Executives in any one organization like to hear from prominent leaders who have good things to say about their organization's employees. I must add, however, that people granted membership in influential networks must be careful to return favors. If they don't, they will be labeled as users and takers and will be banished from the company of prominent individuals.

But how do people develop good networks? One way is to go to various meetings where influential individuals might be in attendance (Smith, 1988). These meetings can include receptions for executives, award ceremonies, political fund-raisers, and volunteer activities for charities and other public service organizations. At this point, an advanced social skill comes into play. Some people can go to such meetings even if they do not know anyone who is likely to be in attendance. They can enter a room, introduce themselves to others, strike up lively conversations, circulate among the many guests in attendance, and contribute to the success of the meeting through their colorful presence. Research by psychologists interested in social skills suggests that about 10 percent of people are comfortable attending such meetings (Zimbardo, 1977). This is a low figure, and it indicates that a significant number of people are uncomfortable developing networks if they have to interact with strangers.

There is certainly criticism of people who develop networks in this manner. Some observers dismiss these activities as glad-handing and schmoozing (Felker, 1969). These observers have often not been the beneficiaries of socially skilled strangers who come up to them and offer introductions to others at various gatherings of prominent community leaders. I find myself in agreement with the critics on one point, however. The development of very high-level social skills can be overdone if it takes away from other skills that people should acquire. People need to develop various abilities such as marketing, computer literacy, organizational skills, and leadership. If they only have high-level social skills, they may be eventually dismissed as intellectual lightweights who only know how to attend social gatherings. My students often ask, "What's more important, what you know or who you know?" I answer that they must keep both in mind. People's various work-related abilities are their "what," and they offer these to the job market. Their networks are their "who," and these are the people who will decide whether they can use the abilities that job seekers present.

Making Others Feel Special. If people have good social skills, they are able to meet strangers and put them at ease. Socially skilled people can discuss a variety of issues and consequently can find one or two topics that are of interest to the strangers. They can disagree with others on important issues without becoming tense or hostile during discussions. When others think of who should be invited to important meetings that will be attended by prominent individuals, socially skilled people top the list.

Some social skills are possessed by a relatively small number of people. One is the ability to make others feel unique and special. Take the simplest example. A person with this advanced skill is having a conversation with someone at a social gathering. The socially skilled person listens carefully, gives careful thought before responding to the other individual's statements, and seems to forget that there are other guests at the gathering. The individual who is the target of this focus and attention feels special and experiences an increased sense of self-worth because of the conversation (Brislin, 1991).

People demonstrate the opposite of this social skill if they have the reputation for "suffering fools badly." When some people meet others who are not particularly well read on a topic or are unprepared for serious discussions, they may dismiss the others as not worthy of their time. These less socially skilled people are unwilling to endure the unpleasantness of keeping up a conversation with someone who has little to offer. One of my colleagues and I were recently discussing skills useful in the business world, and he referred to an individual we both know. My colleague said, "Not only does he suffer fools well, he makes the other person feel like the smartest individual in the world. And, he does all this in a smooth, gracious manner and so has a widespread reputation for working well with many different kinds of people."

Earlier in my career, I worked in Washington, D.C. One of my bosses advised me to watch Senator Edward Kennedy if we were ever at the same reception or political gathering. "He'll move around the room quickly," my boss said, "but the moment he gives any person is seen as special. Further, all people will feel that if Senator Kennedy only had some more time, then he would have chosen to spend it with them and not with others at the gathering." Television commentators discussed this aspect of Senator Kennedy's political skills during tributes to him after his death in August 2009. Judging from the video tapes I have seen, Governor Arnold Schwarzenegger has this talent for "working a room" and making guests feel special.

This advanced social skill is similar to a talent possessed by some entertainers. When I was a teenager, I traveled to Japan with my parents. We saw an elaborate production of the musical "Hello, Dolly" at one of the large Tokyo theaters. Mary Martin played the lead role. There were over 2,000 people in the audience, but when she sang I felt all her attention was directed at me. I'm sure others in the audience had the same feeling.

Working through Taboo Topics Surrounding Networking. There are professional organizations, such as the Academy of Management, whose members meet to discuss behavior in the workplace. At a recent meeting I attended, a session dealt with career development in various countries: Russia, Ukraine, China, Israel, New Zealand, Great Britain, Canada, and the United States. One interesting theme is that people on the road to successful careers need to deal with taboo topics. That is, they need to deal with issues that are extremely important but that are not talked about very often. In addition, when the issues are touched on, many people are reluctant to discuss them fully.

For example, people seeking successful careers in Great Britain need to know about the country's social class structure (Rothton, 2008). However, many British people are unwilling to discuss social class and will even deny its importance. When confronted about the differential treatment of graduates from Oxford and Cambridge compared to an urban public university without a long history and without world-famous graduates, people will avoid the topic and will use generalizations such as, "You can get a good education at lots of schools." There is a similar taboo topic in the United States. Are some people members of elite groups whose members have more access to powerholders and more influence than others? Americans do not enjoy admitting to the existence of elite groups whose members have special privileges (Zweigenhaft & Domhoff, 1991). Such an admission would contradict the value expressed in the Declaration of Independence that "All men are created equal." One of the Americans at the Academy of Management session told others that he went to Harvard and that he belonged to this university's alumni club in Salt Lake City, Utah. He admitted that it is a prestigious club where many of the city's movers and shakers meet to discuss important policy issues in government, business, and academia. In addition, when Harvard graduates travel, there are similar clubs in America's big cities where they will be welcomed as important guests.

Discussions about another taboo topic dealt the assistance that well-established and powerful individuals can offer to people who are developing their careers. In all cultures, there are influential people who can offer or withhold assistance through the sharing of insider knowledge, connections, and invitations to important meetings (Smith, 1988). People who are developing their careers must learn that skills, job knowledge, and a willingness to work hard are not enough. They must also develop connections with powerholders. In other words, they must nurture an influential group of people (the "who they know") so that they can demonstrate their knowledge and skills (the "what they know").

In some cultures, this requirement is captured in vocabulary terms. Roughly translating as one's contacts with important people, Chinese has the term *guanxi* and Russian has the term *blat* (Butler & Purchase, 2004; Gu, Hung, & Tse, 2008). These bear a similarity to an English speaker's network of people among whom favors are given and received. Attendees at the Academy of Management session agreed that an American's networks are easier to develop than the rough equivalents for Chinese and Russians. Americans can develop networks through community activities, evening courses at colleges, and through attendance at professional seminars where they can meet and interact with others. Young Chinese and Russian nationals who are developing their careers are much more dependent on the connections that have been passed on to them by family members or by powerful people who happen to take an interest in them. The ability to develop their own networks through their own efforts is one reason why ambitious people from other countries immigrate to the United States so that they can develop their careers.

WORKING TO DEVELOP SOCIAL SKILLS

A large number of social skills have been discussed in this chapter. These include developing networks, showing respect for others, listening carefully, reacting to criticism without becoming defensive, and making others feel valued in the workplace. Any of these social skills can be improved if people are willing to put in the necessary time and effort. Improving the problematic habits of a lifetime, such as not listening carefully to people, will not change easily. Such habits can be as strong as those that lead to overeating, smoking, the avoidance of exercise, and the misuse of alcohol.

Formal programs for social skills development offered by counselors and professional trainers often have five components (Brislin & Yoshida, 1994). These are information on the rationale for skill improvement, modeling, practice of new behaviors, feedback from others, and transfer of training from the practice site to people's actual lives. Even if people don't have access to formal programs, they can borrow aspects of these five components and can apply them in self-directed efforts for skill improvement. We'll examine the social skills of listening carefully to others and showing respect when others contribute to workplace discussions.

If people want to improve their social skills, they usually are aware of good rationales for their efforts. Socially skilled people are sought out for interactions in the workplace. Because of these interactions, they find out important information about developments that can help them contribute to company goals. Promotions and salary increases can follow. For the second component, modeling, people can try to identify individuals who seem to possess the desired skills and then make efforts to identify exactly what these others do. For example, these socially skilled models might direct all their attention at people who speak up at meetings. They have facial expressions that demonstrate interest. They do not engage in behaviors such as slouching in their seats, staring out the window, or looking at their watches.

Then, people interested in skill development should practice the behaviors they have identified (Martin, 1999). They can practice at meetings associated with their church membership, youth sports if they help with their children's teams, and volunteer work in their communities. The fourth component may be the hardest: seeking feedback. They have to tell friends that they want to make certain changes and need to be told whether they are being successful or not. They might tell friends, "I want to be seen as paying careful attention when others speak during meetings. I'll admit that in the past I would show bore-dom if a speaker was saying things that everyone already knew. If you think my mind is wandering at this meeting, please give me a kick under the table!''

In the final component, people bring the new skills they have been practicing back into the workplace. They show enthusiasm at their organizations' meetings and listen carefully when others make contri-butions. Occasionally, they should compliment people who make espe-cially good points. If people are conscientious about their new behavior, these will eventually become their well-practiced habits (Martin, 1999). In the past, people may have had the habit of looking out the window during meetings. Now, their new socially skilled habit is to give their full attention to others when they speak and make contributions.

9

Attitudes in the Workplace

Job satisfaction, or lack of it, is an important attitude that people bring to their workplaces every day (Boswell, Schipp, Payne, & Culbertson, 2009; Doest, Maes, Gebhardt, & Koelweijn, 2006). Attitudes refer to people's positive or negative reactions to various aspects of their lives (Petty et al., 2003). When any one aspect is considered, it is called a social object. Examples of these objects are one's job, neighborhood, outdoor activities in one's community, and the public schools that are supported by taxpayer dollars. Objects can be seen and touched, and examples of attitudes toward objects are types of automobiles being considered for purchase and brand names of clothing that might be worn to work. Concepts refer to social projects that are more abstract, and often cannot be seen, heard, or touched, but they are nevertheless very important in people's lives. Concepts often refer to ideas that reflect a person's values and self-image. Examples are the types of careers that people want to have and the types of schools to which they want to send their children.

Attitudes contain three components: people's evaluations of social objects, their thoughts and cognitions, and their actual behaviors (Petty et al., 2003). The evaluative component refers to people's overall feelings about a social object. Using the example of people's jobs, the evaluative component would be assessed by asking people how good or bad their jobs are, how positive or negative they feel, and how favorable or unfavorable their experiences have been. If people feel generally positive about their jobs, specific negative experiences are often dismissed as temporary difficulties that can be easily overcome. But if they have an unfavorable evaluation, the same difficulties can be seen as additional specific examples of why the jobs are terrible.

The cognitive component refers to people's thoughts, beliefs, and opinions. This component can be measured by asking people to describe their jobs as objectively as they can. They would then describe their job duties, salaries, coworkers, and other aspects of their work that come to mind. Another way of describing the cognitive component is that it summarizes what people think "the facts" are. People may be wrong, but their overall feelings of job satisfaction are influenced by their perceptions of the facts. For example, their salaries might be very good compared to individuals holding similar jobs in other companies. But if people think they are underpaid, this could affect their job performance.

The behavioral component refers to people's overt actions and activities. These behaviors can be observed and noted by others (Baumeister, 2005; Illies, Fulmer, Spitzmuller, & Johnson, 2009). Do people come to work on time and stay until the end of workday? Do they take a number of sick days that seems excessive? If people are working in retail sales, do they approach and offer help to customers within 10 seconds of seeing them looking at merchandise? Do they meet deadlines set by company executives, or do they constantly ask for extensions? Given that behaviors are overt, they have a major impact on people's reputation among their colleagues.

Distinctions among evaluations, cognitions, and behaviors have been captured in people's everyday language. Individuals may talk positively about a social object, such as the desirability of maintaining contact with customers concerning their long-term satisfaction with the company's products. They may have positive feelings concerning this goal (evaluative), and they may be able to give reasons that it is a good idea (cognitive). These components are different, however, from "walking the talk." People have to actually follow through with their evaluations and cognitions and engage in the behavior of contacting customers who have made purchases in the past.

ATTITUDES AND THEIR IMPORTANCE

People's attitudes help them to organize the incredible amounts of information to which they are exposed. If they have well-developed attitudes about what sorts of work will interest them, they can analyze information about various organizations and be much more efficient in their job searches. If they have well-developed attitudes about food preferences, they can be selective about the advertisements they read that describe the offerings at various restaurants. If they have well-developed attitudes about the topic, "what a good boss does," they will work hard for some of their managers and will minimize their interactions with others (Sherif et al., 1965; Zimbardo & Leippe, 1991).

The field of attitude change has long been studied by both psychologists and communication scholars. Conclusions drawn from some of the research on change may have given the impression that attitude change is relatively easy. Researchers would measure people's attitudes. Then, they would present well-argued facts arguing a position different from people's recently assessed attitudes. They might add other factors to the communication, such as having the facts presented by a high-status individual or by a young but highly experienced person. After listening to these presentations, researchers would measure attitudes again and many people would show that they had changed (McGuire, 1985).

One difficulty with these studies is that they dealt with attitudes about which people did not have strong feelings (Sherif et al., 1965). Given that people did not care too much in the first place about the attitudes being assessed, it did not take much effort to encourage them to change their positions. Examples of topic areas studied in this research were "the importance of getting a regular tetanus booster shot," and "the music of Teddy Conklin, old time vaudeville singer." Discussions of these topics did not cause very many people to experience adrenaline rushes and to shout at others who disagreed with them, in sharp contrast to topics such as publicly funded health care. Another issue was "whether or not freshmen should be able to own and park cars on their college campuses." This was not a hot topic for college students who were sophomores, juniors, and seniors.

When people have well-developed attitudes about which they have strong feelings, attitude change is very difficult. Rather than expect a 180-degree turn from their initial positions, a more realistic goal is to nudge them to examine different concepts relative to their initial attitudes. Let's look at attitudes toward various jobs as examples. If people have a negative attitude about meeting strangers, they may avoid jobs in sales since they will have to constantly meet potential customers and clients. Attitude-change efforts will rarely result in such dramatic change that people actively seek out strangers at company receptions and at social events in their neighborhoods. A more realistic goal is to encourage people to learn techniques for becoming comfortable with meeting new people. They may accept a communication presenting arguments that this skill will likely help them in their quest for job promotions no matter what their position in a company. Understanding the difference between strongly held and weakly held attitudes is important. One way I think about strong attitudes is to ask and answer the questions, "What attitudes will cause people to come to public meetings, such as city council meetings? What will motivate them to leave their homes, give up their normal leisure time activities, and come to a hearing or to a demonstration?" In many American communities, examples are fluoridation of water, limits on the number of cars that people can own, and the placement of garbage dumps. And, of course, there is that golden oldie, regulation of handguns owned and used by individuals. People have intense attitudes concerning these issues, and they do not change easily (Petty & Brinol, 2008; Sherif et al., 1965; Zimbardo & Leippe, 1991).

Weak and Strong Attitudes. People's attitudes can range from weak to strong. Weakly held attitudes might include whether or not politicians should provide financial support for a new modern art museum featuring local artists. While some people feel strongly about this issue, many people don't care very much one way or the other. Some of these uncommitted people can be encouraged to change their attitudes if proponents of the museum make convincing arguments. Such arguments can include how the museum will improve the quality of life in the community, how it will attract tourists, and how it will provide educational opportunities for artistically inclined schoolchildren.

The most effective arguments will match the interests and concerns of people whose attitudes might be changed. People whose jobs are dependent on the visitor industry will pay attention to arguments that a new museum will attract more tourists (Beyer et al., 1997). Parents with school-age children may find that arguments about educational programs for youngsters are compelling. Good communicators are skillful at reading audiences and tailoring their arguments to the interests and concerns of listeners.

In contrast to attitudes about which people do not have strong feelings and thus can be moved in the direction of a speaker's recommendations, some attitudes are very strongly held. These attitudes often are part of people's self-images that they are very proud to communicate to family members, friends, and coworkers. Such attitudes often deal with deeply held values such as the proper role of government in improving community life, religion, and the legal status of a woman's right to an abortion. These attitudes do not change easily and speakers advocating change will find their task to be challenging (Zimbardo & Leippe, 1991). If they advocate for change at community meetings, speakers will be interrupted and will have to deal with angry voices and with audience members who attack both their personalities and their motives.

These strongly held feelings and opinions are sometimes referred to as ego-involved attitudes (Sherif et al., 1965). They are attitudes that are central to people's views of themselves, the types of individuals they are and want to be, and the images that they want to present to others in their communities. Examples of these attitudes that are often in the news include publicly funded vouchers that can be used at private schools, efforts to decrease commute times to work during rush hours, and the choice of sites for public transportation stops.

People often draw from their ego-involved attitudes when speaking out in public forums such as legislative hearings, public demonstrations, and school board meetings. Since the attitudes are deeply held and since they are confident enough to voice their views in public, they will not be easily swayed by speakers who have differing views. Attitudes cannot be captured by a single point on a scale ranging from "disagree very much" to "strongly disagree." Especially for ego-involved attitudes, people have positions that they find acceptable, positions about which they are neutral, and positions that they find unacceptable. If strongly held attitudes are to be changed, communicators must ask whether their message is consistent with at least one position that audience members find acceptable or about which they are neutral. This is a very difficult task for communicators, and helps explain why attitude change regarding important issues is so challenging (Petty & Brinoll, 2008; Petty et al., 2003).

Ego-Involved Attitudes. People have attitudes toward many social objects and concepts, ranging from the very important to unimportant. Attitudes that people hold strongly often deal with very important issues in their lives, such as religion, political affiliations, and careers. These are called ego-involved attitudes because they contribute to people's views about themselves and the public images that they want to present to others (Sherif et al., 1965). Attitudes that are weakly held do not include the element of centrality to people's self and public images. For example, in the 2005 movie *The Weatherman*, the character played by Michael Caine had a very weak attitude toward the music of Bob Seger. He may have hummed along when he heard Bob Seger songs on the radio, but he did not have strong feelings one way or another. He became much more interested in the music when his son quoted from the Seger song "Like a Rock" at a testimonial dinner. The son said that the song reminded him of his father. Michael Caine's character then went to a music store to buy a CD that included this song.

Ego-involved attitudes are not well summarized by single marks on a measuring scale ranging from "like very much" to "dislike very much." Most people have completed measuring instruments of this kind. Managers rate their subordinates on how well they are doing their jobs (Kinicki & Williams, 2008). In doing so, managers are communicating their attitudes about their employees. Audience members at public lectures are sometimes asked to fill out a questionnaire whose purpose is to evaluate the speaker. Hospital patients are asked to fill out questionnaires about the quality of care they received before, during, and after their recent operations (Haskard, Williams, DiMatteo, Heritage, & Rosenthal, 2008). Customers in restaurants are asked to evaluate the service they received.

When people do not have strongly held attitudes about these issues, they have few problems filling out these questionnaires. But when the attitudes involve their sense of self, they can be frustrated because the questionnaires do not delve into the complexities of their views (Baumeister, 2005). In the example of the operations at the hospital, for instance, people may have very strong views that cannot be summarized by a series of marks on a questionnaire. They may have felt that physicians disrespected them by not answering questions about the operation, but they may have found that the nurses gave excellent care. They may have been upset at the number of drugs that the physicians prescribed after the operation, perhaps feeling that they were not adequately counseled about postoperative pain, weakness, and lack of mobility.

The measurement of important, ego-involving attitudes has to go beyond checkmarks on a scale. These attitudes involve what are called latitudes of acceptance, rejection, and neutrality (Lambert, Chasteen, Payne, & Shaffer, 2004; Sherif et al., 1965). Let's use the example of attitudes toward bosses in the workplace. Latitudes of acceptance refer to behaviors about which employees have positive feelings. These might include feelings about the importance of bosses communicating a vision of the future, communicating openly about workplace issues, and giving feedback on how employee work can be improved.

Latitudes of rejection refer to behaviors that employees feel contribute to poor and ineffective management. These can include addressing employees using a demeaning tone of voice, not setting and communicating high workplace standards, and failing to follow through on promises to employees. Latitudes of neutrality refer to behavior about which employees do not care one way or the other. This aspect of attitudes is especially difficult to analyze because some employees will place a behavior in their latitudes of acceptance. Others will feel a behavior is relatively unimportant and will place it in their latitudes of neutrality. Such behavior might include a manager's ability to give ceremonial speeches at company banquets or a manager's participation in voluntary community activities during weekends. The fact that some people are neutral and others are highly positive is one reason for the adage, "You can't please everyone all the time."

Changing Ego-Involved Attitudes: Anticipate Difficulties. Strong attitudes allow people to communicate public images to others. In the business world, strong attitudes can deal with the value of hard work, the importance of giving back to the community through volunteer work, and the necessity of mentoring younger employees. When people hold strong attitudes, they do not change quickly and easily. People who are in favor of unlimited oil drilling do not read Rachel Carson's book, *Silent Spring*, and suddenly run for the presidency of the Sierra Club. Or, they do not read a newspaper article about the dangers of speeding on the freeways and then write to their legislators about the wisdom of installing cameras on freeways to record driver behavior. If people want to address the attitudes of others, a goal more realistic than change is to nudge them to consider different viewpoints and to encourage expansion of their thinking (McGuire, 1985; Petty et al., 2008).

Let's use the example of mentoring younger and less experienced employees in the workplace. Managers may be concerned that young workers are floundering around on the job because they do not know company policies and do not know how to develop new projects. The managers may ask some older and experienced employees to develop mentoring relationships with the younger workers (Borman, 2004; Farh et al., 2008). The potential mentors may object. They may say, "I think I have enough on my plate already. I think I would be neglecting my current projects, and my longtime customers and clients, if I took on mentoring responsibilities."

If managers want more mentoring activities, they have to engage in attitude change. They have to convince potential mentors that time spent with younger employees is good for the company. But, as discussed above, attitudes do not change easily. Managers are well advised to nudge people slowly toward new behaviors rather than to expect overnight change (McGuire, 1985). One step managers can take is to encourage potential mentors to engage in active thinking about the proposal. William McGuire (1985) calls this encouraging the generation of related cognitions. If efforts to influence attitudes are to be successful, people must think about how the managers' mentoring proposal relates to them, personally. That is, they must generate related thoughts or cognitions. These cognitions will be different for different people, and they will often deal with answers to the question, "What's in it for me?" Some potential mentors will consider the thought that if they are successful, younger employees will be able to make more contributions to the company and so ease everyone's workload. Others will think about the possibility of younger employees becoming highly successful in 10 years and then remembering their mentors from the old days. Still others will accept the managers' proposal out of short-term self-interest, feeling that it will increase the chances of their own promotions in their company.

Managers should realize that different potential mentors will accept their proposal after considering different cognitions. They can assist the acceptance of their mentoring proposal by covering a series of ideas in their communications: the spreading out of workloads, the fact that some mentees today will be executives tomorrow, and the types of company activities that look good in promotion applications. Without the generation of related cognitions (McGuire, 1985), potential mentors will shift their attentions from the mentoring proposal to the many other issues competing for their time and efforts in the workplace.

Implications Resulting from Attitude Measurement Issues.

Attitudes are often measured on a scale where people make a mark corresponding to their feelings. For example, they are asked to think about a big company such as General Electric and to rate it on a scale ranging from "very good" through "no opinion" to "very bad." Although convenient and efficient, this measuring technique does not capture the complexity of attitudes (Kinicki & Williams, 2008). It does not capture the richness of people's feelings on issues such as the reliability of General Electric products, follow-up services, the quality of the company's leadership, and the attractiveness of the company as a place to have a career.

Especially for people's important and self-defining attitudes, a better approach to measurement is to examine a wide range of positions. These various positions are organized according to people's latitudes of acceptance, rejection, and neutrality. Let's use the workplace example of managers' attitudes about communicating with employees. For traditional managers who view themselves as the sources of knowledge and authority, the latitude of acceptance (Sherif et al., 1965) will include statements such as "tell employees what to do" and "make sure that employees know what my goals are." These are the communication practices that traditional managers find to be acceptable. But knowing only acceptable practices does not allow for an in-depth understanding of attitudes.

The latitude of rejection may include practices such as "listening to the concerns of employees," and "requesting input from workers concerning decision making in this company." These are the practices that traditional managers will reject, causing workers who want to see more openness in communication to face a stone wall. For some communication behaviors, managers will have no feelings one way or the other, so these practices will be put into their latitude of neutrality. Such practices may include "talking informally with employees out of the office at company parties," and "responding to worker inquiries via e-mail."

Research by communication scholars has revealed an important find-ing that is useful for people who want to encourage attitude change (Sherif et al., 1965). If a recommendation for change falls in people's latitude of rejection, it is often perceived as more negative and more unacceptable than the change agents intended. If the change agents want more participative management where bosses seek out recom-mendations from workers, managers will react to the fact that this is in their latitude of rejection. Part of their reaction will be that they feel they are being criticized and that their authority is being questioned. The individuals requesting the change may not have had such inten-tions. They simply wanted more opportunities to give managers their suggestions (Pencavel, 2003; Strauss, 2006). These strong reactions after placement of suggestions into managers' latitudes of rejection help explain a common workplace problem. Workers wanted change and communicated their suggestions to their managers. But the bosses reacted in a very negative manner. The workers then think, "We had no idea that management would react in such an intense way. We just wanted more workplace communication and a two-way flow of information."

In this example of workplace participation, employees will have more success with attitude-change attempts if they frame their sugges-tions in terms that fall into their managers' latitudes of acceptance or neutrality. This recommendation requires that workers know their bosses well. Such knowledge of others is always useful and important in attitude change attempts. If managers interact in a relaxed manner with employees at company social gatherings, perhaps employees can suggest a weekly informal gathering over coffee where ideas can be shared. Or, if managers enjoy responding to e-mail, perhaps several employees can send separate e-mails with the same suggestion for workplace improvement.

In all such communications, workers should not be demanding and should not threaten their boss's authority. If they fail to take this advice and are seen as overly aggressive, then the boss will dismiss them and will reject their suggestions (Park, Levine, Westerman, Foregger, & Orfgen, 2007).

SOME SPECIFIC ATTITUDES OF IMPORTANCE FOR WORKPLACE SATISFACTION

Up to this point, I have discussed attitudes in general terms, with special attention given to attitudes that are important to people's social identities and to views of themselves. I will turn now to reviews of more specific attitudes that are central to the theme of this book: find-ing happiness at work and avoiding feelings of dread as the workday approaches. Feelings about self-esteem are closely related to people's attitudes that contribute to their social identity.

Attitudes toward Oneself. Self-esteem refers to people's attitudes about themselves. People with high self-esteem feel that they are worthwhile individuals, have resources that they can offer to others, and can make important contributions in their workplaces. People with low self-esteem feel that they are unimportant individuals, that they have little to offer, and do not have the ability to deal with the most difficult tasks in an organization (Neustadt, Chamorro-Premuzic, & Furnham, 2006; Sedikides & Gregg, 2008).

People with high self-esteem project self-confidence and accept challenging work assignments that, if completed successfully, will put them on the fast track for raises and promotions. People with low self-esteem avoid challenging tasks and stick to the routine aspects of their jobs. They communicate to others that they are not very ambitious and that others should not rely on them.

For most people, self-esteem acts like a thermostat (Baumeister, 2005). Growing up in New England, a thermostat was a familiar household feature. On the same day, cold temperature could signal that the thermostat should increase the heat. But if the sun came out and the house became too hot, the thermostat would turn off the heat and might even turn on the air conditioner. Self-esteem serves a similar function as people relate to others. So many benefits in life are dependent on our relations with other people that self-esteem includes estimates of how others are reacting to us. If people act in a boastful or pompous manner, others will react negatively. Because everyone wants to be accepted by others, people with adequate self-esteem will pick up these negative cues and can make changes in their behavior. If the same people are mildly depressed and act in a dour manner, others will see this and will send signals that the people should "cheer up."

Some people can have self-esteem that is too high (Diener, Lucas, & Scollon, 2006). These people are so self-confident and so conceited that they don't notice the negative feedback coming from colleagues. In effect they are saying, "I am already so good that I don't need to pay attention to the much less able people that I have to put up with in my workplace." The result, however, is that over time these people irritate others in the workplace to the point that they are excluded from informal communication channels. Because few coworkers talk to them, they become ignorant of workplace developments that can have impacts on their job performance.

It is interesting to ponder the question, "Where can we find people with extremely high self-esteem?" One answer is "prisons"! Some individuals feel that they are so smart that they can commit crimes because stupid policemen will never catch them. Or, they feel that they are so outstanding that laws against white-collar crimes such as insider trading or misusing public funds should not apply to them.

If self-esteem is measured on a 10-point scale, ranging from "extremely high" to "extremely low," a score of about eight could be ideal. This score is high enough to allow people to bounce back from adversity and to face life's challenges in a confident manner. But a score of eight allows just enough self-questioning so that people are sensitive to others and have the self-insight to realize that these others have much to offer (Diener et al., 2006; Diener, 2009).

Attitudes toward Money. People's feelings about money and the relationships among money, career success, and life happiness are best introduced by means of a short example.

Examinations of Money and Life Happiness Are Complex

After 30 years of hard work, Jack McGuire looked back on his life. Now 55 years old, he could point to many accomplishments. He was president of a company that employed 300 people. His own income amounted to $250,000 a year. He drove a nice car, lived in an upscale neighborhood, and was counted among the movers and shakers in his community. But he felt no great sense of personal happiness. He said to himself, "I don't feel any happier than when I was working my way through college delivering pizzas in a rattletrap Ford."

Jack is facing a dilemma experienced by many successful people. He has money and status markers showing that he is highly successful, but he doesn't feel much happier than he did when he was scraping by in a low-paying job. The old cliché, "Money doesn't buy happiness" should certainly come to mind. But the lack of a direct relationship between money and happiness is only part of a complex picture (Diener & Diener, 1996; Kesebir & Diener, 2008).

Up to the point where money leads to the purchase of life's necessities, there is a direct relationship. That is, as people earn enough money to buy a house, pay their utility bills, purchase food, buy clothes for their children, and own a reliable car, they become happier. The opposite is especially true. If people don't have enough money to provide food and shelter for themselves, or to buy clothes for their children that are comparable to those worn by their classmates, they experience stress and unhappiness. But once they are comfortable providing the basics for themselves and their families, additional money is no guarantee of increased happiness.

One reason for this lack of increased happiness is that people's comparison levels change. Jack, for instance, probably experienced pleasure when he was able to ditch his old Ford and buy a reliable Honda. But given success in his mid-fifties, he may experience the revolution of rising expectations. In his social circles, a Honda may not seem like much. To keep up with his peers, he may have to purchase a Mercedes, a Porsche, or a BMW. But keeping up with his peers may not bring additional happiness since he is meeting the expectations set by others, not necessarily doing something meaningful and important to himself. The experience is similar for housing. He may have been proud when he could purchase an apartment 25 miles from his workplace. But with success, he may feel pressured to purchase a home in an expensive neighborhood closer to theaters and museums in the city where he lives. Dealing with such pressures may not be important for his feelings of happiness (Kesebir & Diener, 2008).

The pursuit of money and success, as in Jack's experience, can have additional downsides. He may have spent so much time and effort expanding his business that he neglected to nurture family and community social relationships. He may feel that his business success was accompanied by so much stress that his health has been threatened (Lazarus, 1991).

For many people, seeking and achieving balance in their passions and activities can contribute to increased happiness (Triandis, 2009). Balance means that people are giving attention to their work as well as to their interpersonal relationships. Balanced people also find time for hobbies, physical activity, a good diet, medical attention when needed, and volunteer work for charitable activities that they feel are important. Successful executives often tell colleagues that if their success allows them to "give back to their communities," then they feel that their hard work has been worthwhile.

Attitudes and Behavior. The complex relationships among money, career success, and happiness are reminders that the study of human behavior often reveals seeming inconsistencies. A related inconsistency is the well-researched finding that people's behaviors are not always consistent with their expressed attitudes (LaPierre, 1934; Olson & Maio, 2003).

Actions Do Not Always Follow from Words

"As we expand our product line, I'd like to do some market research to see if there are enough potential customers for our new offerings," Sharon Chung told her staff. Sharon was a manager in a company that marketed software programs for home computers in 12 retail outlets. One product in which she was interested was a publishing program that would allow people to write their own books with most of the features of professional printing companies. The program would also allow people to price and to market their books using password-protected Web links. The projected cost for the program was $200.

Sharon asked her marketing staff to prepare a questionnaire that would be administered to a wide variety of people. "Lots of people feel that they have had enough life experiences to write a book, and I believe they will be able to do so using this software." The marketing staff followed Sharon's wishes. After analyzing the answers to the questionnaire, the staff reported that a large number of people said that they would buy the software. The people were also quick to describe the topics they had in mind for the books. These included life on a minor league baseball team, growing roses in Hawaii, improving the public school system, and the history of the banjo. Sharon decided to sell the publishing software program in her company's retail outlets. However, the program sold poorly and Sharon's bosses expressed their disappointment.

The decision to market the software program was based on people's intentions as expressed on a questionnaire. Sharon has encountered a common problem in predicting people's future behavior. What people say they will do is not necessarily what they will actually do (LaPierre, 1934; Olson & Maio, 2003). This is captured in the expression that "some people walk the talk." That is, for some people, if they talk in a certain way, they can be depended on to follow through. People who only "talk the talk" become known as windbags who are full of empty promises.

Why is there a disconnect between what people say and what they do? One reason is that it is easier for people to talk about what they want to do than to behave in ways that are consistent with their intentions. Imagine a running event where people have to go over hurdles. Just about everyone can jump over hurdles that are 12 inches off the ground. But fewer people can smoothly jump over hurdles that are 40 inches high. Expressing intentions on a questionnaire is like traversing the 12-inch hurdles. It is an easy task. Actually behaving according to one's intentions is like jumping over the 40-inch hurdles (LaPierre, 1934).

Another reason for the disconnect is that people are not always skillful at analyzing future situational pressures that may interfere with their intentions (Zimbardo & Leippe, 1991; Zimbardo, 2007). When engaging in the easy task of responding to the questionnaire, they don't think of reasons that would interfere with writing a book. These reasons include finding the necessary time, obtaining the necessary permissions if material is to be cited from other books, overcoming the writer's block that occasionally bedevils all authors, and responding to stories from friends about acquaintances who lost thousands of dollars trying to publish their books. Before actually spending $200 for the software, people begin to think about these potential problems for the first time.

Professors in business schools sometimes use a joke to communicate the difference between stated intentions and actual behavior. Four frogs are sitting on a log that is floating in a pond. The four frogs declare that they are going to jump into the water. How many frogs are there on the log? The answer is four because talking about a jump into the pond is not the same as actually doing it.

Self-Perceptions. If people recognize difficulties and then make efforts to change relevant attitudes and behaviors, they often develop a new view of themselves as individuals who no longer are hindered by their past difficulties (Baumeister, 2005).

The Influence of "That's the Sort of Person I Am"

After working with new college graduates who entered his company over the last 10 years, Mike Doherty finally decided that he needed to learn more about information technology and desktop computers. Now 60 years old, Mike had gone to college during the days of mainframe computers housed in a special building on campus. Given that computers were not in every college building—never mind not on everyone's desk—he had used the mainframe only for special projects. Mike observed that the recent graduates were very computer-literate and that their skills helped them in their work. They were able to do research on potential customers and clients that helped in the development of business proposals. They used their computers to create documents and could deliver "camera ready" manuscripts to printers. Recent graduates could summarize empirical information on Excel spreadsheets and integrate compelling graphics into PowerPoint presentations. They were even able to write their own programs that met the specific needs of day-to-day operations.

Mike decided that he did not want to be viewed as a workplace dinosaur and as a person who was out-of-date regarding the changing workplace. So Mike decided to enroll in a nighttime community college course called "Information Technology for Beginners." The instructor introduced various computer skills to class members, always showing patience when people did not understand how to use a certain program. After six weeks of the class, Mike felt that he was making good progress. After 12 weeks, he began to use his new knowledge when working on various projects in his workplace. He decided to sign up for a second and more advanced course at the community college.

About halfway into this second course, he knew that he was learning a great deal when one of the recent college grads came to him and asked a question about importing video clips from the Internet into a PowerPoint presentation. After about a year, Mike found that he was able to keep up conversations about information technology with all his coworkers. He was now an enthusiastic supporter of computer use in the workplace and recommended new software programs to company executives.

Mike has benefited from an attitude-change process known as changing self-perceptions (Bem, 1972; Ashmore, Deaux, & McLaughlin-Volpe, 2004). The change proceeds along a series of steps. People try a new behavior with which they were previously unfamiliar or which they found distasteful. Outcomes stemming from the new behavior are positive. People then say to themselves, "These new behaviors led to positive results. I guess I'm the sort of person who can perform these behaviors and can reap the benefits. I'll keep performing the behaviors." In Mike's case, his positive self-perceptions lead to the desire to increase his computer skills. The new behaviors that people perform should be voluntary, not forced. People can be nudged and encouraged, as Mike was on observing the computer skills of younger coworkers, but actions should stem from free will. The behaviors should lead to successes.

Good educators, workplace trainers, and career coaches know this and take steps to ensure that students and protégés feel that they are making progress. Further, people going through attempts to change their behavior should be able to demonstrate improvements that they can see in themselves. When people publicly demonstrate their new behaviors, as Mike did in his workplace, there will be even more reinforcement when people observe the positive reactions of others.

The power of positive self-perceptions can be used for many types of behaviors. The person who starts losing weight by eating only salads at lunch may see the results after standing on a bathroom scale. The person can then say, "I'm the sort of person who can lose weight successfully." The person may then adopt other weight-loss behaviors such as exercising and cutting down on high-calorie snacks between meals. Or, people who had the reputation as being loners in the workplace can have lunches and coffee breaks with others. If those others request help, the people can develop the self-image of "I am a person who is asked for assistance on difficult tasks. That's the sort of person I am" (Baumeister, 2005).

10

Decision Making

Part of every manager's job is to make decisions that affect various stakeholders that occupy and surround an organization. One of many applicants must be selected for a job. One employee, but not another, will be given a promotion. One area of the country will be served through company expansion, but not another. Some products and services will be retained and others will be eliminated. The number and importance of decisions that have to be made are often major criteria in establishing executive compensation packages.

Decision making can be done quickly using conveniently available information and tried and tested precedents from the past (Chu, Spires, Farn, & Sueyoshi, 2005; Weber & Johnson, 2009). Such decisions are often called "off the top of the head." Other decisions are made after careful information gathering and painstaking deliberation (Ferreira, Garcia-Marques, Sherman, & Sherman, 2006). Unfortunately, both types of decisions can lead to organizational malfunctions. The topics of this chapter include quick and relatively effortless decision making, the careful and effortful consideration of well-researched alternatives, and problems that can plague many different types of decisions in organizations.

QUICK DECISION MAKING: HEURISTICS
AND PROBLEMS BROUGHT ON BY BIASES

Many times, decisions should be made without large amounts of time and effort involved in the process. Managers have to develop the talent of identifying problem areas that lead to quick recommended solutions and problems that are worthy of the costs associated with careful deliberation (Tversky & Kahneman, 1973; Weber & Johnson, 2009).

Heuristics. Heuristics refer to "rules of thumb" that quickly come to mind when people are expected to make decisions (Hogarth & Karelaia, 2007; Tversky & Kahneman, 1973). Often, heuristics are summarized in adages or short phrases that are commonly shared by members of a community.

Informal Rules of Thumb Guide to Workplace Decision Making

After accepting the presidency of a video production company, Alice Chandler met with individual employees for a series of one-hour exchanges of information. She wanted to get to know her 40 employees as individuals and to learn their recommendations for company policy in the future. After two weeks, she called her first meeting of all employees. One of her recommendations was, "Whenever you have a problem that requires my attention, please see me as soon as possible before difficulties get out of hand. I agree with my mother who frequently talked about a stitch in time saving nine."

If Alice is using the adage that a few stitches today will prevent bigger problems tomorrow, then she is using a heuristic in her recommendations to her employees. Heuristics are informal rules of thumb that give guidance to decision making (Tversky & Kahneman, 1973). Some heuristics are summarized in adages. I have heard Chinese businessmen say that "You can't eat a char siu bao (a large meat-filled bun) in one bite." The businessmen are pointing out that large projects have to be broken down in smaller components. Other heuristics are used because they are easily available to people and can be drawn quickly from their memories. After terrorist attacks in the United States, people became much more concerned about airport security because the dangers of travel were vivid in their minds (Triandis, 2009).

People use heuristics to guide their decision making when they do not have time to do research on all alternative possibilities. Given people's busy schedules and multiple demands on their time, shortcuts to decision making are commonly used (Hogarth & Karelaia, 2007; Kahneman & Tversky, 2000). If businesspeople from Hawaii have to stay overnight in Los Angeles on their way to Memphis, it is not a good use of time to do research on all possible hotels. People are likely to use heuristics such as "near the airport" and "part of a chain of hotels I have stayed at before where the room was satisfactory." The quest to find an "excellent" rather than a "satisfactory" hotel room is not worth the effort for most business travelers. Similarly, people do not have time to do research on all places to have a business lunch. They are likely to use informal guidelines such as,

"My friend, who has good taste in food, recommended it and the restaurant has lots of parking."

Sometimes people are the unwitting victims of heuristics. When reviewing applications for employment, hiring officials sometimes examine whether or not applicants have given all the information that has been requested. Hiring officials have told me that they view incomplete applications as coming from incomplete people. The officials do not have time to interview 40 applicants for one position. If they pare down the number to be interviewed based on completeness, they are using a heuristic in their decision making.

A commonly heard heuristic takes its toll on businesses in Hawaii. When the American economy is not doing well, leading to lower tax revenues, county officials from many parts of the mainland United States cancel their reservations for previously scheduled conferences in Hawaii. In the past, the media have picked up on the fact that there would be a convention here, and many stories and TV spots predicted that county officials would bask in the sun and skip important meetings. In this and related cases of "paradise avoidance" when people have serious conventions or business dealings in mind, Hawaii is the victim of facile heuristics (Erev, Glozman, & Hertwig, 2008; Goldstein & Gigerenzer, 2002). People are very busy and face many decisions on a daily basis. These include decisions about workplace improvements, service to customers, votes for political candidates, education for the community's children, time and money for the support of churches, and so forth. In a perfect world, people would have infinite time to make decisions about these issues (Simon, 1978). They would have the time and energy to research the issues, list pros and cons of many possible choices, and attach weights to various options corresponding to their importance. With all this information, they would be able to make careful, highly rational decisions. But the world is not perfect. People simply do not have enough time for this type of careful decision making.

Instead, people rely on heuristics (Hogarth & Karelaia, 2007). These guidelines to quick if imperfect decision making are also known as "rules of thumbs." Heuristics often can be summarized in memorable phrases or images that come quickly to mind. People then recall these phrases and images when it comes time to make a decision. Instead of reading every review before going out to a movie, a person can say, "Roger Ebert gave it three stars." Instead of studying every make and model before purchasing an automobile, a person can remember the advertisements that featured several enthusiastic locals talking about the respect they received at a certain dealership. Instead of considering all options for entertainment at a preschooler's birthday party, a person can remember the heuristic that "kids always like clowns who can make balloon animals."

Hawaii can be the victim of heuristics when people in other parts of the world make decisions that involve the economy of the state. What comes to mind when people think about Hawaii? The answer is some variant of "sun and fun," with related images such as surfers paddling out to the big waves and sunbathers lolling on the beach. This is a tough heuristic (Fiedler, 2000) to fight when residents of Hawaii invite people to come here for serious conventions or high-level business discussions. The people who would come to Hawaii have difficulties communicating with others in their communities. They are almost certain to hear something like the following from their friends and work colleagues: "You're going to Hawaii for a convention? Yeah, sure! I bet you'll go to lots of meetings! I'll check the quality of your tan when you get back!"

People are well advised to know the heuristics that may be used negatively against them. I frequently discuss this issue when advising my students from Hawaii who are seeking jobs on the mainland. I advise them to be very careful when preparing their resumes. Hiring officials who read resumes may immediately think of the fun and sun metaphor and immediately conclude that applicants from Hawaii cannot have the seriousness of purpose that successful careers demand. For this reason, students from Hawaii should emphasize their accomplishments that will be attractive to hiring officials. What advanced certificates have they earned? What club activities did they lead? What internships did they complete during which they impressed executives? To what specific company goals can they attach their talents? Applicants from Hawaii should take pains to combat the fun and sun heuristic and to replace it with another in the minds of the hiring officer: "From reading this resume, I think that this applicant matches my view of what this company needs."

Adages. I was discussing heuristics and decision making with my business students recently and was surprised that some of the adages that I learned many years ago are no longer well known. When I discussed the advantages of working with the same company for many years, students did not know the adage, "A rolling stone gathers no moss." When talking about identifying problems before they become threats to the organization, they were unfamiliar with "A stitch in time saves nine." When discussing the advantages and disadvantages of risk taking when starting new business ventures, they did not know the old saying, "A bird in the hand is worth two in the bush." The students certainly know the concepts captured by these heuristics, but they were not familiar with the exact phrases that I learned during childhood.

So what adages do business students in Hawaii know? One heuristic with which they are very familiar is "What goes around comes around." I believe this is a well-known adage because Hawaii is a relatively small community and people who live here want to stay. They realize if they engage in behaviors that have a negative impact on others, then those behaviors will be remembered and will come back to haunt the perpetrators. Further, since relationships are so important in Hawaii, negative behaviors are not limited to one targeted person. The behaviors will affect and will be remembered by the victim's extended family and by close friends. And people have very long memories. Negative behaviors from 20 years ago can be treated as if they occurred yesterday.

This adage becomes part of advice concerning ways of dealing with difficult people. I remember being in a conversation with businesspeople and lawyers. One person complained about the abusive behavior of an executive in Hawaii and wondered what might be done about it. A lawyer replied that one approach would be to wait for the executive to become the recipient of the ill will he has generated. "I've also heard of this executive," the lawyer continued. "His negative behaviors will come back and take their toll."

Often, the same advice can be captured by different adages that become shared among people who speak the same language and live in the same part of the world. One equivalent to "what goes around comes around" is "you reap what you sow." If people cause too many difficulties and contribute to a stressful workplace, their behaviors resemble seeds that gardeners put into their soil. Later, difficult people will find themselves the recipients of the ill will that grows from the seeds that they planted.

Biases: The Escalation of Commitment. A major reason people use heuristics in decision making is that time is a precious resource (Weber & Johnson, 2009). If they can make decisions on topics where a satisfactory decision is appropriate ("Should we stay at Holiday Inn or the Marriot on our next business trip?"), they will have more time to invest in decisions concerning more difficult topics. The investment of various resources often leads to predictable biases in decision making.

People invest various types of resources in their pursuit of life happiness. Although the most frequently discussed resource is money, there are others that play a major role in people's decision making. People invest the important resource of time in their formal education, deciding that years spent in college will pay dividends at a future date. They invest energy in voluntary activities hoping that they can contribute to a better quality of life in their communities. They work hard to acquire specialized knowledge in areas that will advance their careers. For all these decisions, there are opportunity costs. Money, time, and energy spent on one set of activities means that those resources are not available for other attractive alternatives.

In addition to problems of opportunity costs, people have a difficult time knowing when to stop their investments of resources (Hsee &

Rottenstreich, 2004). They have difficulty saying to themselves, "This activity in which I have invested is not paying off with any benefits. It is time for me to cut my losses and move on." Instead, people often continue to invest their resources, hoping that outcomes will turn out better. The problem is called *escalation of commitment* by behavioral scientists who study real-life decision making. Instead of admitting that their original decisions were poor and led to losses, people often escalate their commitment to their decisions. They run the risk, then, of losing even more resources in attempts to gain back their original investments.

The problem can be seen in the workplace. Some people are unhappy with their jobs (Iyengar, Wells, & Schwartz, 2006). But given that they have spent so many years to prepare themselves for success in those jobs, they are reluctant to cut their losses and seek other types of employment. They may be unhappy in the accounting profession, for example, but they are concerned with their previous investments. They may have spent four or five years in college, and in addition may have invested in internships and in additional coursework necessary to become certified public accountants. Instead of changing careers, they might say to themselves, "If only I give accounting a couple more years, maybe my day-to-day work will change and be more enjoyable." In making this decision, they rarely consider the possibility that those additional years will then form an additional commitment to accounting that will make it even harder to change in the future.

The escalation of commitment can be seen in the vacation plans of many people who enjoy gambling in casinos (Denrell, 2007). They go to Las Vegas and, like most people, lose money. But instead of cutting their losses and making other types of vacation plans, they plan their next trip to Vegas. Part of their decision making often includes the heuristic, "Maybe I can win back the money I lost on my last trip."

The refusal to recognize and to cut losses is a widespread problem. It can occur in relationships. Consider two people who have been a romantic item for five years. The relationship is not terrible, but neither is it so positive that it contributes to the happiness of the two people. Friends and family members comment that the relationship seems to have problems, and the two people know that they have more spats than they should. But do they cut their losses or do they escalate their commitment? Many will escalate and will say, "Let's give this relationship six more months and maybe it will turn around for the better." If they make this decision, they will not have those six months to meet other people with whom they might form more satisfying relationships.

ATTENTION TO CAREFUL DECISION MAKING

Whenever people make important decisions, there are always both positive and negative aspects. Even when a decision seems likely to lead to only positive outcomes, there can be unforeseen difficulties. If nothing else, the time, energy, and resources devoted to one alternative decision cannot be applied to another possibility. If people travel to another city for two weeks of job interviews, for example, they cannot spend this same amount of time contacting members of their networks for information about job possibilities in the community where they currently live. Once important decision areas have been identified and people know that they want to move beyond simple heuristics, formal decision making can help (Chu et al., 2005; Simon, 1978).

Strengths, Weaknesses, Opportunities, and Threats. Making a list with two columns, one for positive and the other for negative aspects of a decision, is a good starting point. The outcomes of such a list can be the basis for a SWOT analysis (Kinicki & Williams, 2008). This acronym is derived from the first letter of four issues to be addressed when considering alternative decision possibilities: strengths, weaknesses, opportunities, and threats. Strengths refer to personal or organizational features likely to lead to positive outcomes. For job applicants or people seeking promotions, strengths include education, work experience, successful project completion, and skills that executives will find useful. Weaknesses include skills and abilities that executives desire but which applicants do not possess. In my experience working with job applicants and people seeking their first promotion, these include a lack of public speaking experience, limited computer literacy, and the inability to disagree with others without being strident and unpleasant when presenting their attitudes and opinions.

Opportunities refer to possibilities that allow personal or organizational growth. If a state's economy is improving and more companies are seeking opportunities, then there are clearly opportunities for people seeking employment. Alternatively, people may decide that given their strengths, they will find more opportunities if they travel out of one state and settle in another. Threats refer to real or imagined barriers that can interfere with the pursuit of opportunities. Too often, threats are self-imposed by people who are convinced that they can't improve their skills and will be stuck in their current positions. Employment counselors often encourage people to identity their strengths and to use these to combat the pessimism that too much focus on self-limiting threats can bring. If they can move from pessimism to optimism, they can focus on real threats such as competition from others for employment and promotions (Seligman, 1991).

People can often use their strengths and predicted opportunities to address their weaknesses and perceived threats. For example, people may recognize that one of their strengths is the ability to learn material quickly. If they also feel that one of their weaknesses is the inability to speak a second language, then they can use their strength and take language courses offered by a university's outreach program. If they feel that they are good communicators but lack computer literacy, they can take evening courses or can buy self-teaching tutorials on such skills as the use of PowerPoint, statistical analysis using Excel, and Web design. Later, they can combine their ability to communicate effectively with their newly developed computer skills. They can let executives know that they not only can use computers, but also can help other employees with whom they would work. Whether they are seeking their first jobs or a promotion, this combination will be a new strength that will differentiate them from their competition.

Avoiding Stereotypes. Often, careful decision making involves careful and deliberate attention to cognitive biases (Chapter 2) and other threats to informed thinking. People have a strong tendency to form stereotypes of others based on age, ethnicity, gender, nationality, medical condition, and a host of other factors (Allport, 1954; Hyun, 2005; Risen et al., 2007). Careful decision makers downplay the temptation to stereotype. When I give presentations to members of various organizations, this issue arises. Members of workshops I offer often begin with a question such as this.

"You've talked about differences in behaviors that take place in Hawaii compared to other parts of the world. At my company, we want to hire more local people rather than import them from the mainland. Do you have any advice for us?"

I have complex feelings about giving advice because I know that my perspective involves a stereotype. Anytime individuals make generalizations about a group of people, they are entering the strong possibility of stereotyping members of that group. The individuals should be uncomfortable with their thinking, as I am when making recommendations about the desirable goal of hiring more locals. But if I keep my advice to myself, will I do more harm to locals than if I give my recommendations?

The stereotype is that locals are not as talkative and verbally expansive during job interviews (Bernstein, 1971; Howard, 1964). When asked a question, many locals will answer it with a terse seven- or eight-word statement. People from the mainland, competing for the same jobs, will answer with a much longer answer and will do so with a more animated tone of voice. There are certainly exceptions to this generalization, and we can see them in the worlds of business, entertainment, education, and social services. But so many employers have shared this stereotype with me that I believe it has some reality, if nothing else than in the heads of people who will make important hiring decisions.

So I share the generalization with hiring officials. I then offer other advice. I suggest that they look carefully behind the answers of locals and mainlanders. Just because mainlanders use 30 words, this does not mean that they are saying more than locals who use 10 words. Another piece of advice is to give people preparation time. I advise employers to allow all job applicants to prepare themselves. This can be done by sharing questions before the actual interview. Locals can be very verbal and expressive if they have time to think about and to rehearse various types of presentations. The stereotype of "the quiet local" comes from a discomfort with speaking up on the spur of the moment, even if there is nothing to say. Mainlanders (remember, I am including myself here!) are much more comfortable filling empty time with talk.

Nancy Adler (2002) has also wrestled with issues surrounding people's use of stereotypes. Realizing that people will stereotype no matter how much they are told not to, Adler suggests that they can become more sophisticated in their thinking. People can learn to view stereotypes as a first best guess about a person. They discover various labels that can be applied to a person, such as "local," "mainlander," "Republican," and "professor." Then, they can be open to movements away from the stereotype as they gain more specific information about any one person from the stereotyped group. People can constantly caution themselves that they should not make decisions based on stereotypes and should allow others to communicate and to demonstrate their unique abilities and personalities.

Using Statistics. Of all of the courses students take in college, one of the most unpopular is statistics. Students in many disciplines suffer through a required course and sometimes plan a lighter load in other areas to make sure they have sufficient time to pass statistics. Disciplines that require one or more courses include business, education, psychology, sociology, nursing, medicine, and agriculture. Even though they may be the kindest and most cooperative members of their departments, statistics professors are often unpopular with students and become targets of their cynical humor.

Reasons for unpopularity include mathematics anxiety, and this problem would apply to other required courses such as calculus. Another reason is that the use of statistics asks people to go beyond their initial impressions after they casually examine an important issue. People spend years learning to form first impressions, and often their conclusions are good enough to deal with issues in a satisfactory manner. Statistical tools can give more information than initial impressions, but these tools must be mastered in a relatively short time compared to the years people have relied on their gut reactions.

The use of statistics can reveal problems of which any one individual is unaware. Faye Crosby (2004) has argued that women often underestimate biases in the workplace that put them at a disadvantage. If one woman has not been the target of bias, or if she dismisses biased behavior as a temporary aberration, she may decide that her organization is supportive of women. But if an informal survey is taken where many women respond, basic statistical analysis may lead to the conclusion that the organization has problems. If 30 women are questioned and 12 give examples of biases, this is a trend that management should examine. Other statistical tools can determine if the biases are reported more in one department compared to another, whether specific executives are involved in more than one example, and if older women report more problems than younger women.

If careful efforts to gather information from many employees are not undertaken, there may be a misperception known as "false consensus." If nobody speaks up publicly about biases, people may conclude that the organization has no problems (Gendolla & Wicklund, 2009). People may not complain individually because they remember their mothers' admonition, "If you can't say something nice, don't say it." This can be especially true in small communities where social norms include the additional guidance for everyday behavior, "Don't talk behind people's backs."

Good managers should go beyond informal conversations and casual impressions (Janis, 1982) and circulate questionnaires asking about problems, suggestions for improvement, what customers are saying about the company, and so forth. Analysis of the results will often identify actions management should take to improve the organization so that it attracts the most able employees.

INEVITABLE DIFFICULTIES IN THE DECISION MAKING PROCESS

Whether decisions are made with the help of heuristics or careful thinking, people will inevitably encounter a number of predictable consequences. Even if the decisions are carefully reached and well-intentioned, there can be troublesome outcomes for example, once people make a decision, they want to justify it as wise (Festinger, 1957; Connolly & Zeelenberg, 2002).

Post-Decision Dissonance Reduction. The strong tendency to justify the quality of decisions can be seen in this incident.

People Justify Decisions through Complex Thought Processes

The hiring committee at an import-export firm narrowed the candidates for a managerial position to two people: Steve Kim and Andrea

Tanaka. Both had excellent qualifications including advanced university degrees, enthusiastic letters of recommendation, and relevant job experience. But the committee could select only one person. One member joked that he held their resumes up to a light to see if he could assess the quality of the paper on which the two candidates had printed their resumes. The committee members finally settled on Andrea. Right after the final polling of the committee, members felt relieved that they had made the right decision. Andrea was clearly the better candidate, and they wondered why they considered Steve for such a long time.

The committee members may be justifying their difficult decision through a process called *post-decision spreading of alternatives*. This process is part of cognitive dissonance theory (Festinger, 1957; Connolly & Zeelenberg, 2002). When people make important decisions, they need to justify them to reinforce their own positive self-images and to communicate to others that they are good decision makers. They can achieve these goals by thinking of reasons that justify their decision. This elaborate thinking is especially important when people have more than one alternative about which they have to decide. Once they decide on an alternative, there is cognitive dissonance since they might be making a mistake. "Perhaps the other alternative was better, and I will look like a fool for making the wrong choice!"

The decision whether to smoke or not is a good example. People may say to themselves, "I smoke, but it would improve my health if I decided to stop smoking." The people will be in a state of cognitive dissonance if they consider that their decision to smoke may be hazardous to their health. So they must justify their decision to maintain a favorable view of themselves. They can do so by dismissing the research linking smoking to health difficulties. Or, they can point to self-perceived benefits of smoking, such as weight control or stress reduction.

In the hiring case, dissonance arises from the possibility that the committee made the wrong choice between two attractive candidates. One way for committee members to reduce the dissonance is to spread the alternatives (Festinger, 1957). The positive points of Andrea's background are emphasized, and the negative aspects of Steve's resume and experience are highlighted. If they engage in this elaborate thinking, committee members may feel much more confident when they make their recommendation to the firm's executives. Because the executives will see only the post-dissonance rationale for the recommendation, they are likely to read about Andrea's successes and Steve's shortcomings. This decision-making process can work against the firm in the long run. If executives recognize the reality of dissonance reduction, they may offer the job to Andrea but will not dismiss Steve from their minds. Rather, they will keep in contact with him in case there is a future job opening for a highly qualified candidate.

Pluralistic Ignorance. When large numbers of employees who might have input into decisions do not share their views, executives might conclude that a consensus has been reached (Halbesleben, Wheeler, & Buckley, 2007).

Silence Does Not Mean That Everyone Understands What Is Being Discussed

Having called a meeting of her senior management team, Allison Scruggs summarized a consultant's report to the 12 people in attendance. She began, "As you know, we called in a consultant to do a study of worker motivation and morale. The consultant concluded that the well-known distinction between self-evaluation and self-efficacy is central to understanding motivational issues in our company." Allison then paused to see if there were any questions or comments. People glanced at each other and each individual wondered if he or she was the only person who did not know the distinction between self-evaluation and self-efficacy. But since no one wanted to admit to this lack of knowledge, nobody spoke up. Allison then continued the meeting, having concluded that everyone knew what she was talking about.

Allison has encountered an example of pluralistic ignorance (Halbesleben et al., 2007). No one person wants to admit that they don't understand the terms that the boss is using. In reality, nobody knows the distinction to which Allison was referring. But because no one asks a question, the boss feels that everyone is on the same page. So the meeting continues with everyone ignorant of what is being discussed. If Allison continues her discussion of workplace motivation, the company meeting will be a waste of everyone's time since there is no understanding of the concepts being discussed.

Self-evaluation refers to general assessments people make of themselves (Baumeister, 2005). People with a positive self-evaluation view themselves as worthwhile individuals who have a great deal to offer to their workplaces and to their communities. People with high self-efficacy view themselves as competent to perform specific workplace tasks (Osman-Gani & Rockstuhl, 2009). Different people feel self-efficacious about different tasks. Some salespeople, for example, feel that they are better at contacting potential new customers than they are at closing deals.

People can have positive self-evaluations but can also admit that they have little self-efficacy with certain workplace tasks. Senior executives who are proud of their career accomplishments can marvel at the sophisticated computer skills of recent college graduates. They can be excellent executives without negative feelings of self-efficacy about their clumsiness using sophisticated software.

To combat pluralistic ignorance, someone at the meeting has to sense that many of the attendees do not understand the concepts being discussed. That same person then has to speak up and ask the boss to clarify the terms being used. Often, others will later thank the person who spoke up, saying, "I thought I was the only one who did not understand, but I noticed that everyone was paying very close attention when the boss explained the terms that she was using." The unwillingness to speak up and ask basic questions is undoubtedly one reason why people dread going to meetings in the workplace. No one wants to admit ignorance and so meetings drone on without a shared understanding of the ideas that people are supposed to discuss (Halbesleben et al., 2007; Janis, 1982).

Although the term *pluralistic ignorance* is recent, the psychological phenomenon it captures is not. In Hans Christian Andersen's tale, "The Emperor's New Clothes," two con artists convinced the head of state that they had a beautiful suit that they wanted to sell him. The suit would be invisible to him because he was so intelligent, but common folk in the kingdom would admire it. So the king paraded down the street in his skivvies, and everyone cheered since they did not want to admit that they could not see the suit. A young lad finally spoke up, "The emperor has no clothes," thus contributing a phrase that has long since been used to puncture pomposity.

Parkinson's Law. When he was host of television's *Tonight Show*, Johnny Carson tried to ensure that the show would have large amounts of unrehearsed and spontaneous behavior. He felt that audiences liked to see the unpredictable in his interactions with his guests and in his responses to on-the-spot groans after unsuccessful jokes. Given this preference, rehearsals for a *Tonight Show* episode might take no more than one hour. A reporter once asked him, "Why don't you increase rehearsal time for each show? I should think this would make for better-prepared guests, better sound for the musical acts, and more jokes that audiences find funny." In his response, Johnny Carson used just two words: "Parkinson's law."

This law describing human behavior, formulated by Cyril Northcote Parkinson, states that work expands to fill the time available (Parkinson, 1957). In the case of the *Tonight Show*, Johnny Carson felt that he could put on a good show with one hour of solid work during rehearsal. But Parkinson's law states that if there were six hours of rehearsal, the same amount of work would expand to fill this larger time slot. People would slow down their normal pace of work. They would rehearse musical numbers three or four times, but would not notice-ably improve the final product. More jokes would be tried out, but the resulting collection would not be funnier.

Put another way, there would be a great deal of "busy work" added so that six hours of rehearsal time would be filled. Executives would probably hire another assistant just to schedule time slots within six-hour rehearsals. Johnny Carson felt that the strong possibility of busy work, and a person to supervise it, would be poor use of resources and so kept to the one-hour rehearsal policy.

There are examples of Parkinson's law in many types of organizations (Brannon, Hershberger, & Brock, 1999). A colleague told me recently of a meeting of her church's advisory board. She said, "There was only about a half-hour of work to be done. But the meeting was scheduled to run for two hours, and so the full two hours were filled. People brought up issues and old stories that had nothing to do with the current administration of the church." Given their social skills, people might not show boredom and displeasure during the two-hour meeting. However, they might invent a convenient excuse and avoid coming to the next meeting, fearing that it would be a poor use of their time.

Recently, Parkinson's law has been applied to information technol-ogy, especially personal and office computers (Bryce, 2006). It reminds people that the use of computers becomes more inefficient as storage space increases. When people have large amounts of storage space, they become careless and expand the information they choose to keep. Useless e-mail messages from five years ago are not deleted but instead are saved. Teenagers' computer games that they have outgrown still take up storage space. People do not take the trouble to learn how to use efficient data compression programs since there seems to be no limit to what they can store. Similar to the *Tonight Show* possibility, organizations sometimes have to hire a computer specialist to help peo-ple manage access to their constantly expanding data.

The Peter Principle. If people perform with distinction in their cur-rent positions, there is no guarantee that they will perform well if they are promoted to higher positions (Peter & Hull, 1969).

The Peter Principle: Why Do Organizations Have So Many Problems?

"I think it's time we gave Matt a promotion," the vice president of an insurance firm told other executives at their weekly meeting. "I have in mind that he will supervise all agents in our life insurance di-vision." Matt Bartlett had been one of the most successful salespersons in the company. He had consistently placed in the top five agents based on policies sold each year, had opened up areas of the city where the firm had previously been unsuccessful, and had a good reputation for follow-up service with clients. Only one of the executives at the meeting had reservations. She said, "I hope we don't fall prey to the Peter Principle with this promotion."

This principle of bureaucracy, formulated by Laurence Peter, states that people in an organization will be promoted to their level of incompetence (Peter & Hull, 1969). The principle assists in answering the question, "Why doesn't anything work very well around here?" People are hired in an organization and perform well in their entry-level jobs. Some are promoted, even though their new jobs involve skills that they did not necessarily demonstrate in their entry-level positions. This process of job performance and promotions continues until people take positions where they demonstrate incompetence. Because of their poor job performance, they will no longer be candidates for promotion. However, it is very difficult to demote employees in a bureaucracy, especially if their jobs have union protection. So, according to the principle, managers and executives in an organization eventually take on jobs where they will perform poorly.

Although formulated with a sharp sense of humor, this principle does seem to capture the career development of people who had good reputations prior to poor performance in their current positions. In Matt's case, for example, there is no guarantee that the skills he demonstrated as a salesperson will lead to good performance as a supervisor. As a sales agent, he would develop good networks in a community, approach clients, tailor his sales message to the different needs of clients, and so forth. As a supervisor, he would participate in the selection of agents, would oversee their training, and would make judgments about subordinates' progress in their work. There is no automatic carryover from skills demonstrated as a sales agent to those needed as a supervisor. Matt may find himself in a position where he cannot demonstrate satisfactory job performance.

Even though there are no guaranteed solutions, the dangers of the Peter Principle can be addressed if executives recognize potential dangers. One approach is to use situational interviews when making decisions about promotions (Noe et al., 2008). Matt would be asked to place himself in situations likely to arise if he became a supervisor. An executive might ask, "What would you do if you received several complaints about the follow-up service provided by one of your salespeople?" Or, "If you identify a specific reason an agent is doing poorly, such as difficulties in closing sales, what would you do?" There are no automatic correct answers, but executives could judge whether or not Matt has thought about such questions and if he is prepared to move from excellence as a sales agent to excellence as a supervisor.

The Importance of Specific Examples of General Issues. What do the following issues have in common?

- The dangers of smoking and the wisdom of kicking the cigarette habit
- Preparations in California regarding decisions made today for natural disasters that may occur in the future
- The proper role of government and its impact on people's everyday lives
- The reality or the myth of global warming and the power of people to have an impact on their environment.

All of these issues are very important and should be discussed frequently. However, the issues are rarely discussed unless there is a current, specific example that directs people's attention and stimulates them to converse with others (Brislin, 2008; Kahneman & Tversky, 2000; McGuire, 1985; Zimbardo, 2007). In the smoking example, scientists have known for years about the dangers of cigarettes. However, people are much more likely to discuss this topic if there is a celebrity who recently died from a disease related to smoking. Recent discussions of smoking, together with widespread promises to give up the habit, occurred after the death of ABC news anchor Peter Jennings. In the case of preparations for natural disasters, people asked what the local government has been doing after coverage of hurricanes Katrina and Rita. We should not have to be reminded about the importance of proper preparations given past experiences over the last 100 years with destructive storms, but people seem to need specific examples to stimulate them to action.

The proper role of government will always be a hot topic for conversations (Brislin, 1991; Crick, 1982; Crosby, 2004). Should there be more government programs aimed at addressing problems? Or do government programs create bloated bureaucracies whose members are more interested in looking good than in solving problems? This issue is currently under discussion in light of the perceived effectiveness or ineffectiveness of the gas cap law. Should government become involved, or should marketplace forces be allowed to operate unhampered by imposed price limits? Global warming will become the topic of conversations as a possible contributor to the number of hurricanes along the Gulf Coast.

Other issues will be discussed, such as hurricane cycles that occur every 30 or 40 years. Hopefully, these conversations will also stimulate examination of what people can do to improve their environment through their own actions. Such actions include finding alternatives to fossil fuels, more attention to the recycling of paper to reduce dependence on forests, and the proper disposal of hazardous chemicals to cut down on pollution.

People need specific examples of complex topics. If they try to discuss issues in the abstract, they begin to sound like groups of individuals who are often chided for being very boring. These groups include academics, armchair philosophers, and (described with a mild sneer) intellectuals. In addition, examples need to be current. In discussions of governmental decision making, examples such as van cams to catch speeding drivers could be brought up. But this issue, a hot topic several years ago, would make a speaker seem quaint and out of date if it were discussed today. If people in Hawaii start talking about the preparation for evacuations in the event of a hurricane, they may come across as worrywarts and alarmists if there has not been a major storm in the last five years.

When I was growing up in New England, one of the adages that people used was, "Don't lock your barn door after the horse has been stolen." The time to lock the door is before someone might come into a barn to steal a horse. More generally, the adage reminds people to prepare today for problems that may occur in the future. Although the advice to prepare for problems in the future is wise, people seem to need the experience of losing a horse before they take actions to prevent future losses.

THE IMPORTANCE OF SITUATIONAL
FACTORS ON DECISION MAKING.

One of the themes covered in several chapters is to understand the importance of the forces people experience as they interact in various social situations. Behavior is not just a result of people's personalities, preferences, and attitudes. Rather, people are sensitive to the situational cues they observe and unconsciously sense in their day-to-day social interactions (Blass, 2004; Brislin, 2008; Zimbardo, 2007). I would like to examine this theme as it assists in the analysis of decision making. Let's examine decision making regarding how best to interact with bosses.

Employees want to predict the behavior of their bosses (Kelley, 1967; Moore, 2000; Tetlock, 1985). For example, they ask, "Will my bosses look favorably on this proposal for change? Will they seriously consider my request for a promotion? When they made comments after my last public presentation, were they being constructive or were they showing displeasure?" Most commonly, people assess the personalities of others when they make predictions about behavior. If their bosses are dynamic individuals who are looking toward the future, then employees may predict that plans for organizational change will be well received. Or, if bosses constantly look for ways to improve themselves and feel that employees should be interested in self-growth, employees may take comments about their speeches as constructive criticism.

Although personality is certainly important, behavior is better predicted by combining information about people and the social situations in which they find themselves (Brislin, 2008; Zimbardo & Leippe, 1991). At times, behavior that might seem inconsistent with our knowledge of people is clarified when the pressures of social situations are integrated into our thinking.

This important point can be clarified by an example. Mary is an executive in an insurance company whose duties include supervising sales agents. She was known as an effective mentor who worked cooperatively with both well-established sales agents and new hires. One morning, she had long conversations with two employees. Joe had worked in the company for 12 years and his sales had recently declined. Mary discussed reasons for this decline with Joe and they prepared a plan of action that they felt would lead to improvements. Mary ended the meeting with the comment, "I know that you can do better."

After this meeting, Mary met with Peter, who had been hired six months ago. Peter had not met his sales quota and was performing worse than Joe. Nevertheless, Mary encouraged him, pointed to successful sales that Peter had closed, and told him that he was an asset to the company. She ended the meeting by saying, "Keep up the good work!"

Mary is clearly making different decisions concerning how best to deal with Peter and Joe. But is she being inconsistent? The answer is "no" if we take the perspective that behavior is best predicted through a knowledge of people's personalities and the social situations in which they find themselves (Mischel, 2004). Mary has a people-oriented, cooperative personality. She has the goal of improving sales. With Joe, an established agent, she behaves in one way. With Peter, a new hire, she behaves differently. But the entire picture becomes consistent when we keep in mind that Mary is interacting in two different social situations.

The people with whom we interact are major aspects of social situations (Brislin, 2008). In the first situation, Mary needs to find out why Joe's sales are declining. They devise a plan for improvement. In the second situation, Mary needs to encourage a recent hire. So she focuses on reasons that allow her to offer praise. Her goal of improving sales is best served by adjusting her behavior according to the varying demands she experiences during her workday.

People's behavior that seems inconsistent becomes much more understandable when observers take into account both personality and situational influences. Let's examine two more examples. Beverly is known as a quiet employee who does not enjoy public speaking and rarely voices her opinions at company meetings. But on the weekends, at picnics involving her large extended family, she is lively and animated. She is known as a person who can be counted on to contribute to successful picnics. She is also a good organizer and calls family members to be sure they know about social gatherings.

Ray is a mid-level manager in an accounting firm. His subordinates do not consider him a good boss. He is harsh and demanding, addresses his employees in an unpleasant tone of voice, and regularly criticizes their work in public settings. When he is with high-level executives in the firm, however, he is polite and charming. He addresses the executives in a respectful tone of voice and tells them what a great job they are doing.

The behavior of Beverly and Ray may seem inconsistent because they are not behaving the same way in different social situations. But if person-situation combinations are considered, their behavior becomes much more understandable. These combinations are called *behavioral signatures* by Walter Mischel (2004). Signatures include information about people's personalities and the social situations in which they regularly find themselves. Beverly has a quiet and introverted personality. She does not speak up at company meetings, but she is the life of the party at weekend family gatherings. This is a common signature. Many people become very open and expressive when they are in the company of people whom they have known all their lives. But they are quiet and withdrawn with people whom they don't know well, as is common in many large workplaces.

Ray is harsh and unpleasant with subordinates but seems like a charm school graduate when he is in the company of company executives. This is a common signature of people with authoritarian personalities. Such people are very sensitive to their positions in power and status hierarchies. They often "dump down" on subordinates to demonstrate their self-images of powerful people who have to right to order others around. But they "suck up" to people who have more power and status. Authoritarians want the approval of high-status people and obtain feelings of satisfaction by associating with company executives and other influential people in their communities.

Whenever people ask me to explain puzzling behaviors they have observed, I try to encourage them to think about both personalities and situations. Was a normally pleasant person rude because she was under a great deal of stress on a certain day? Was a normally punctual person late because of a family medical emergency? Did a person who usually contributes to charities turn down a request because of recent financial troubles? Thinking about both personalities and situations is difficult, but it allows for fairer and more accurate analyses of people's decisions regarding their behavior (Kelley, 1967; Mischel, 2004).

11

Worker Motivation

The people a company is able to attract to its workforce will always be its most important asset (Noe et al., 2008). Without a capable and highly motivated workplace, a company cannot provide goods and services, cannot respond to customer demands, and cannot make adjustments in dynamic business climates (Huang, 2008). No matter how talented workers are, however, there is the danger that they will be lulled into complacency if managers do not consistently communicate high expectations and reward excellent performance. These managerial tasks are part of the complex process of motivating the workforce, and I will discuss this topic by examining various theoretical ideas that scholars have developed to explain worker motivation. At the end of the chapter, I will try to provide some integration to the various theoretical viewpoints.

Motivation starts with knowledge of worker valences (Porter & Lawler, 1968; Villere & Hartman, 1990). That is, managers need to know what will move their workers from the status quo to a more ambitious set of company goals. *Valences* consist of what workers value. Workers want an adequate salary so that they can satisfy physical needs for themselves and family members. These physical needs include food, shelter, clothing, and a means of transportation. Once these physical needs are met, people very quickly become concerned with their motives, or what they find personally important in life. *Motives* go beyond physical needs and deal with psychological requirements such as acceptance by others, the opportunity to pursue tasks that are seen as important, and the possibility of helping others achieve their goals.

After managers make sure that their workers have adequate salaries such that physical needs can be satisfied, they need to address psychological concerns (Maslow, 1943). Managers need to know their workers well enough so that they can help employees satisfy their motives. Employees bring a diverse set of personally important valences to the workplace. Some enjoy constant communication with others, sharing what they know, and having numerous positive interpersonal relations with coworkers. Some employees enjoy taking on tasks where they can demonstrate personal achievements (McClelland, 1985). They want to write a training manual, open up new territory for marketing the company's products, or bring in a large number of new customers. Other employees enjoy being in charge of different work groups. They enjoy organizing the diverse contributions group members can make, are good at delegating, and are skillful when giving people feedback on the progress they are making.

Good managers know their employees and can assign them to jobs where they are able to satisfy their motives. Employees who enjoy working with others often find success in a company's human resource division. Or, they may find that they enjoy positions where they are expected to provide long-term services to customers. Managers are blessed if they have employees who enjoy feelings of achievement upon the successful completion of tasks. With these employees, the manager's job is to make sure that the tasks undertaken are consistent with overall company strategy. Other employees may not be able to demonstrate stellar achievements through individual efforts, but they enjoy being in charge of a large work group. In other words, the employees enjoy the feelings of power that are associated with directing the efforts of others (McClelland, 1985; Winter, 1973). Managers need to monitor the work of employees who enjoy positions of power. If left unchecked, some employees will become intoxicated with power and will become abusive toward group members. This will lead to task failure and employee turnover.

Managers must harness the diverse talents that employees bring to the workplace. They must also be clear about workplace contributions that will lead to salary increases and promotions. Managers must also be aware of key distinctions that will have an effect on decisions concerning how best to harness the talents of employees. One important distinction concerns worker motivation and morale.

MOTIVATION AND MORALE

Recently, a manager asked me this question after I gave a presentation to employees at the small business where she worked. "I served on the panel reviewing the yearly evaluations of employees in the organization where I serve as a vice president. One employee was judged to be highly motivated but to possess little morale. Another was said to have morale but little motivation. I think that both employees make important contributions to the organization. What exactly is the difference between these two terms?"

My answer started with the assertion that motivation and morale refer to different types of behaviors that people bring to their organizations (Weakliem & Frenkel, 2006). The distinction lies in the difference between individuals and the groups to which they belong. *Motivation* refers to reactions in the workplace. If people set goals and strive to achieve them, then they are motivated. The goals can reflect their individual interests. Some people have the goal of bringing in the most clients to a business. Some want to provide the best customer service to a relatively small number of clients. Other people want to keep current in their areas of expertise and so buy technical manuals and take evening courses through a university's outreach programs. Success in meeting these goals leads to reputations such as, "This employee works hard and can be depended on to achieve carefully set goals."

Morale refers to people's relation to the organization as a whole and to coworkers. There are always factors beyond any one individual when morale is discussed, and the other factor always involves other people in the organization. People with high morale are proud to work for an organization. When they discuss themselves, they talk enthusiastically about the place where they work. They have positive feelings about coworkers and respect the contributions that others make to the organization (Grant & Mayer, 2009). They are willing to make personal sacrifices for the good of the organization.

If people are highly motivated but show little morale, they benefit their organization through their hard work but not by their contributions to the projects initiated by others. If they have high morale but low motivation, they benefit their organizations by self-sacrificing efforts. They put emphasis on their contributions to their organizations and not to their individual careers. Some people can be high in both. They are hardworking, ambitious, and want the organization's highest-paying jobs. These same people can be cooperative in the workplace, can show respect for others, and can demonstrate pride in their organizations.

The distinction is especially important today. Some people are emphasizing employability (De Cuyper, Notelaers, & De Witte, 2009) rather than employment. They are giving attention to their own skills and are always ready to find a job given the range of contributions that they can offer to a company. They are motivated to have good careers, but feel no special attachment to any one organization. Such people are influenced by their personal experiences, with sudden downsizings imposed by companies, which preached but did not practice loyalty to employees. Many motivated employees will work hard for an organization but will always "have suitcases packed" in the form of cutting-edge skills and good networks that they offer to the job market.

THEORY X AND THEORY Y

One of the most prominent contributions to discussions about worker motivation was developed by Douglas McGregor (1960). The term he developed, *Theory X and Theory Y*, is frequently heard in the business world.

Dreading and Enjoying Work: Two Theories

With her degree in business, internship experience, and active participation in university clubs, Sandra Cronin felt that she was ready for a set of job interviews with various companies in the Pacific Northwest. She discussed her plans with the professor who had taught courses in management and organizational behavior. Sandra discussed various companies where she would seek interviews. Her professor commented, "You have an interesting collection of Theory X and Theory Y organizations. Do you remember the class discussion about the differences?"

Theory X refers to an organization whose executives believe that people don't like to work. Executives believe that people work only as hard as necessary to provide food and shelter for themselves and their families. Given this belief, executives feel they must engage in constant supervision and they try to manage employees with carrots and sticks. They dangle "carrots" in front of people in the form of pay for piecework, overtime pay, or vacation time. Or, they manage behavior with "sticks" in the form of various punishments should employees not perform at the level expected by executives. In Theory X organizations, executives invest little in staff development efforts such as training programs since employees will probably leave the company in a few years.

Theory Y, as explained by McGregor (1960), refers to an organization whose executives believe that people can enjoy work. People can find fulfillment in the workplace and can experience major contributions to general life happiness. A management policy involving only carrots and sticks is not necessary. People will work because they enjoy what they are doing. Certainly a competitive salary and set of benefits is necessary; however, Theory Y executives do not have to spend all their time monitoring employee behavior. Executives can put resources into staff development. They can be confident that their investment will pay off since employees will stay with a company where they enjoy working.

Theory Y can be seen in the behavior of people who clearly don't have to work. Most readers know of people in their sixties and seventies who could retire comfortably. But the people continue to work because they enjoy it. They know that various needs will be met in the workplace: socialization with others, the sense that they are doing something important, and the feeling that they are making positive contributions to others. Winners of multimillion-dollar lotteries often continue working at their same jobs even though they could invest their money and live comfortably.

The terms *Theory X* and *Theory Y* have become so well known that people going through job interviews for managerial positions could encounter them. To obtain information concerning how managers would deal with employees, members of an interview panel might ask about the applicants' views concerning the two theories.

THE DESIRE FOR COMPLEXITY

Often, some Theory X workers want to become Theory Y workers, even if they are unfamiliar with these terms and instead just do not enjoy their work. They may dread getting up in the morning as the first step in the process of going to work. These people may find their work boring, repetitive, and lacking in importance. They would like to be employees who value their work and make important contributions, but they cannot find satisfaction in their current jobs. Managers can sometimes motivate these bored workers by increasing the complexity of the tasks that are assigned to them.

Various factors contribute to enriched jobs that people enjoy (Hackman & Oldman, 1980). The first is skill variety, which refers to the number of different abilities that a person brings to a job so that it can be completed successfully. Service managers at automobile dealerships must have social skills to work with customers, must know technology to work with mechanics, and must have mathematical skills to prepare billing statements. They also have to know the basics of marketing since they have more dealings with the public than other specialists within an automobile dealership.

A second factor contributing to job enrichment is task identity (Saavedra & Kwun, 2000), or the opportunities to complete an entire task or a clearly identifiable piece of work. The classic example of a job with low task identity is an assembly line position where a person repeats the same small chores again and again over an eight-hour workday. Computer technicians have jobs with high task identity. They can enter a company having problems with information technology, can diagnose problems, and can make necessary repairs and adjustments. They can observe the happy faces of people getting back to their computers and using them in their work.

A third factor is task significance, or the impact of one's work on people's lives (Hackman & Oldman, 1980). Elementary and high school teachers clearly have a major impact on the lives of their students. Nurses play a major role in all aspects of a patient's time spent in the hospital prior to, during, and after surgery. Insurance agents contribute to people's financial peace of mind through various policies covering their health care, home, and automobiles. Workers whose jobs involve high task significance would answer "strongly agree" after reading the statement, "The results of my job have a significant effect on the lives and well-being of other people."

The fourth and fifth factors deal with employee decision making and knowledge of how they are doing. Enriched jobs permit workers to be autonomous and to make their own decisions about how to carry out assigned tasks. The number of supervisors needed to oversee workers should decrease as employees become more autonomous. Enriched jobs also allow workers to know what they are doing right and what they need to do to improve their performance. This feedback can come from many sources, including supervisors, customers, and coworkers. It can also come from the job itself, as when automobile mechanics see customers driving away in smoothly running cars that had to be towed into the repair shop a few hours ago.

There is an important caveat if managers decide to move toward increasing job complexity. Job enrichment only is effective with employees who have growth needs (Oldman, Hackman, & Pearce, 1976). Such employees want to improve, want to obtain raises and promotions through their efforts, and want to have the reputation of dependable, hardworking people who value their contributions to their workplaces. Increasing the complexity of jobs will not be welcome by unmotivated and clock-watching employees who come to work only to earn enough money so that they can pay their bills and pursue their hobbies.

MOTIVATORS AND HYGIENES

The distinction between people who want to be known as productive workers and people who just want a paycheck provides a good introduction to the question, "What do workers want?" The answer is not the same for everyone.

Theory X people do not look forward to the start of their workdays. They show up at their workplaces and carry out their assigned tasks only to earn enough money to pay their bills. Or, they try to earn enough money to find life satisfaction in other activities such as hobbies and voluntary community service. Theory Y people enjoy their work and look forward to successful careers (McGregor, 1960). When asked questions about what they would do if they won $10 million in a lottery, many people say they would continue to work. For these people, jobs and careers are a major part of their social identities. They are satisfied with their work, and they are motivated to be good workers.

Various aspects of the workplace, and intrinsic aspects of people's jobs, lead to satisfaction and motivation (Herzberg, Mausner, & Snyderman, 1959). Some aspects do not lead to satisfaction, but they help avoid dissatisfaction (Sachau, 2007). Imagine a horizontal line. At one end there is the phrase "I am dissatisfied with my work." In the middle, there is the phrase, "neutral," or "I am neither satisfied nor dissatisfied." At the other end of the scale, the phrase "I am satisfied with my work" appears. People make a checkmark along this line corresponding to their feelings about their work.

Some workplace issues prevent dissatisfaction. That is, they lead people toward the neutral point on the scale that corresponds to the feeling that "my work is merely okay but I don't get a whole lot of satisfaction from it." These aspects include the quality of supervision, or in everyday language, how good the bosses are. Other aspects keeping people at the neutral point are attractive company policies, physical working conditions, relations with other people in the workplace, and job security. Since they prevent dissatisfaction, they are called *hygienes*. The distinction between "preventing dissatisfaction" and "contributing to satisfaction" can be puzzling. One way I think about it is to recall a television advertisement from years ago. A man was talking about a deodorant. He said something like, "Using this deodorant does not guarantee me an active social life, but it keeps me feeling and looking fresh. And when you think about it, that's quite a lot." The deodorant is like workplace hygiene. It does not guarantee positive outcomes, but it prevents a person from becoming a total social outcast.

With attention to a second set of workplace issues, people can change from neutral feelings about work to feelings of satisfaction and fulfillment. Since these aspects move people to become more satisfied and to look forward to their workdays, they are called *motivators*. These workplace aspects include opportunities for promotion, opportunities for personal growth as unique individuals, recognition, increased responsibility, and achievement. These aspects are more associated with career development over a number of years and deal with more than just a job during any ordinary day at the office. They also deal with features of people's identities as hardworking individuals who have a lot to offer. If good workers do not find these motivators in the workplace, they will often seek employment in other organizations. Managers are wise to examine the list of motivators and to ensure that their companies allow workers to move from the neutral point to job satisfaction.

Readers may have noticed that one very important aspect of the workplace was not discussed in this coverage of hygienes and motivators. That aspect is money. This is such an important issue in the workplace, with implications for both preventing dissatisfaction and contributing to satisfaction, that it deserves special attention.

So where does money fit into the list of motivators and hygienes? In Frederick Herzberg's original formulation (Herzberg et al., 1959), pay prevented people from becoming dissatisfied but did not move people from the center point to actual job satisfaction. More recent research has given money a much more prominent place in studies of motivation. Current arguments are that people's feelings about their pay both prevent the negative feelings of dissatisfaction and contribute greatly to the positive feelings that accompany workplace satisfaction. In fact, if employers can give attention to only one workplace issue, assuring good compensation for the most productive workers is the most powerful step that they can take in their pursuit of organizational success (Brislin, MacNab, Worthley, Kabigting, & Zukis, 2005).

Why has the role of workplace salaries changed from preventer of dissatisfaction to a much more central role in the analysis of workplace motivation and employee growth? One reason is the world economy has changed over the last 50 years. In the past, families could support themselves with the work of one wage earner. During my childhood, for example, my father worked and my mother stayed home and raised four children until we reached our teen years. The family did not live luxuriously, but the children had access to the basic contributors to youthful happiness. But now, most families need two or more wage earners to make ends meet. The lack of enough money at the end of the month contributes to stress when bills cannot be paid and when additional borrowing is necessary. With extra money, on the other hand, people can afford the pursuit of activities that add meaning to life and that offer pleasure. These pursuits can include music, athletics, spiritual activities as people become active in churches, and community service. If people have to hold down two and three jobs, as is common in many parts of the world, they have no time for these enriching activities.

Another reason for past neglect of pay as a motivation is that many researchers felt that the study of wages and salaries was crass. They asked, "Aren't there more important motivating factors that can contribute to people's feelings of transcendence and self-actualization?" Given that people can't seek self-actualizing (Maslow, 1943) experiences unless they can pay their bills, current researchers in the workplace are paying more attention to equitable compensation (Gagne & Forest, 2008). These researchers sometimes quote Albert Camus: "It's a kind of spiritual snobbery that makes people think they can be happy without money."

PREFERENCES, EXPECTANCIES, AND COMPARISONS WITH OTHERS

The treatment of motivators and hygienes provides a good introduction to a complex model of motivation that includes worker preferences for specific types of rewards, such as money, opportunities for growth, and pleasant coworkers. This model then moves into expectancies people have for their workplace, their abilities, their feelings of equity after comparing themselves with others, and subsequent feelings of satisfaction. These multiple ideas are summarized by the expectancy model of motivation developed by Porter and Lawler (1968). We will start with what workers want, also called their valences.

Different Workers Want Different Outcomes: Valences and Rewards. Managers have the responsibility of ensuring that their departments are contributing to company goals. As part of this complex task, they must make sure that workers under their supervision are motivated to work hard and effectively for the company. Motivating the workplace is multifaceted. A key step is that managers must communicate that if employees put their valences to work, then various rewards will come their way.

Valences include people's various psychological requirements. Some people enjoy cordial interactions with many different individuals, and they will be unhappy if they find themselves working alone in an office. Some workers enjoy taking on challenging tasks and basking in the praise that accompanies goal achievement (McClelland, 1985). Some workers enjoy nurturing and helping others. Managers need to make sure that all these different workers understand that if they apply their valences to various company tasks, they will be rewarded. Rewards include salary increases, travel, promotions, advanced training opportunities, and perks such as prestigious parking spaces. Managers can also communicate how punishments can be avoided. If there are three awards to be given out at the yearly company banquet, those not receiving awards may find attendance at the banquet to be punishing. Good managers communicate how to obtain the awards and how to avoid the indignity of never receiving public recognition for stellar efforts on behalf of the company (Eisenberg, 2007; Martin, 1999).

Managers need to make sure that workers feel that there are close links among themselves, their valences, the rewards they desire, and their company. Workers should be able to say to themselves, "I know that I have talents, such as working well with others or working hard on tasks that are assigned to me. I want to be able to use my talents in the workplace. If I am able to employ my talents, then I know that the managers in this company will reward me with promotions and salary increases."

The lack of links between valences and rewards can be seen in many unsuccessful job candidates. Some people do not seem to have valences that can be used in the workplace. They work only because they need enough money to support themselves (McGregor, 1960). Further, they do not seem able to apply any of their talents to the successful pursuit of company goals. In addition, some do not see a link between their own behavior and any rewards that a workplace can offer (Porter & Lawler, 1968). They feel that even if they work hard, nothing good will happen to them (Seligman, 1991). Such people often do not pass a company's initial screenings for new hires. In preparing their resumes, they are unable to communicate that they have talents of use to the company and that they have a good work history where their behavior has led to rewards. Job applicants are advised to use active verbs like "produced, achieved, led, and organized" on their resumes. One reason is to make selection committee members aware that they have talents and know that hard work leads to rewards.

Once managers have identified workers who are confident that application of their valences will lead to rewards, they need to deal with worker expectancies regarding what they can do for the organization. Managers also need to help workers plan for their future in the company.

Employee and Employer Expectations. Another important step in motivating the workforce is dealing with employee expectations. If people are willing to work hard and know that they will be rewarded, then they have a desire to invest their best efforts into the company. But will these best efforts lead to success? Do people have expectations that their hard work will lead to positive outcomes in the future? If they do have such expectations, are they confident about positive outcomes in their current company, or do they feel that they will have more career success if they move to another organization (Porter & Lawler, 1968; Villere & Hartman, 1990)?

Young people's experience with basketball provides a good example of expectations. Many children and teenagers play organized basketball. This satisfies different valences: physical exercise, achievement, and the satisfaction of working with teammates. There are various rewards such as applause from adults, admiration from same-age peers, trophies, and sometimes newspaper coverage. So with the combination of valences and rewards, people have a desire to perform. But what about expectations for the future? Do young basketball players expect to continue with the sport and to attain the riches and fame of professional athletes? Most people conclude that they do not expect to play on a professional basketball team and so look for other career-developing possibilities.

People who gamble or who know gamblers are familiar with another example of expectations (Shead & Hodgins, 2009). Year after year, millions of people travel to Las Vegas, Reno, and Atlantic City with the expectation of going to casinos and winning money. They feel that they can beat the odds, which always favor the casino, and come home with more money than they brought. Even if they come home with less money, they put their positive expectations into planning for their next trip.

When applied to worker motivation, managers must communicate that employees have a positive future. Workers need to know that if they work hard for their present company, then they will have good careers. Workers should be clear about the future possibilities of promotions, salary increases, travel, and other company perks. Managers do not want to lose their best workers. If employees feel that their expectations concerning the future are pessimistic given their present employment, they will likely switch jobs. This will leave managers holding the bag. Managers will have lost good people and will have to go through the time and expense of hiring new workers.

Unfortunately, positive expectancies are no guarantee of success. People must also possess the appropriate abilities to accomplish difficult and challenging tasks.

Employee Abilities. If workers have positive expectations, this means that they are confident concerning a clear link between their needs and motives and the certainty that they will be rewarded if they work hard. Further, they feel this confidence is appropriate in their present organization and do not feel the need to search for greener pastures elsewhere. Problems arise when expectations do not meet various realities that workers may face. People must move from unrealistic fantasies to goals that can be achieved given the resources that they possess and those that can be acquired in the future.

One resource is the abilities that workers possess (Meyer, Salovey, & Caruso, 2008; Moon, 2003). People may expect to do well if they pursue their goals in a certain occupation, but they may not possess the necessary abilities. Coaches and teachers are often faced with the terribly difficult dilemma of counseling young people whose abilities do not meet their expectations. Adults want to encourage young people, but they often have to introduce reality during discussions concerning the level of ability needed for success in various pursuits. Participation in youth sports is a clear example. Young athletes may have the expectations that a Division I scholarship will pay their college expenses. But coaches and teachers often must intervene and caution high school athletes that the competition for college scholarships is intense. For the most selective universities, students must demonstrate both athletic and academic abilities.

To continue with our discussion of gamblers, their interests and efforts provide another example of expectations and abilities (Shead & Hodgins, 2009). Millions of residents travel to various casinos with the expectations of winning a great deal of money. Some feel that they have abilities that will lead to the accomplishment of their goal. They feel that they are good blackjack players, can identity slot machines that are ready to pay off, and have a system for winning at roulette. Many times, their abilities are overwhelmed by the odds that favor the casinos. This reminds me of an old joke. Question: What do casino owners say to gamblers who feel that they have a system that will guarantee big winnings? Answer: "Welcome!"

People can bring various abilities to the workplace. Abilities nurtured as part of people's formal education include verbal skills, mathematics, and a general knowledge of local, national, and world events. People who have the ability to work well with others, also known as social skills (Baron & Tang, 2009; Meyer et al., 2008), will always be in high demand. Other abilities include spatial skills, important in the work of architects and engineers. Physical abilities such as balance, ability, and stamina are important for athletes and dancers. Intrapersonal skills, including the possession of accurate self-knowledge concerning how a person is seen and judged by others, are important for anyone who participates in an organization's marketing activities. Abrasive and self-centered people often do not possess the ability to understand their effect on others (Meyer et al., 2008). These people become unpleasant coworkers, even though they populate the ranks of interesting television reality show participants given the conflicts they generate.

Abilities are not set in concrete at birth. People can develop their abilities as part of their formal education, extracurricular activities during their school years, job experiences, and community service projects. People are well advised to nurture close relationships with teachers, counselors, and mentors who can offer advice concerning skills development. Given good relationships with these trusted advisers, people can ask, "What abilities should I continue to develop given my career goals and expectations?"

Role Clarity. At this point in the analysis of motivated workers, managers are interacting with employees who are willing to work hard, are clear about rewards in their organization, and are taking steps to continue the development of their abilities. Now managers need to make sure that employees can satisfy the role demands of their jobs (Dierdorff, Rubin, & Morgeson, 2009). *Roles* is a term that refers to behaviors associated with a title that people give to themselves and others (Brislin, 2008). There are many titles that can be applied to people: leader, parent, boss, teacher, mentor, computer user, volunteer, coach, teammate, church member, and so forth. There are behaviors associated with all these titles. If people are successful with their titles such as leader, boss, or computer user, this means that they can perform a collection of appropriate behaviors, also known as role requirements. For example, good leaders listen carefully to employees and communicate a clear vision of a better future if workers accept the organization's goals (Yukl, 2010). Good mentors share sensitive and candid information about the organization with younger employees and suggest hands-on experiences that will assist the employees in their pursuit of successful careers (Allen, Finkelstein, & Poteet, 2009). Good computer users solve tasks efficiently and offer assistance to coworkers who are not as knowledgeable.

Managers need to assist workers to meet the role requirements of their jobs (Porter & Lawler, 1968). They can start by making lists of the behaviors that effective workers should be able to perform. Some of these behaviors will demand sophisticated technology, others will involve a great deal of technical information, and still others demand interpersonal skills. For example, many of today's workplaces demand computer literacy. Managers need to provide up-to-date hardware, software, and training. Salespeople need to have cell phones so that current and potential customers can easily contact them. Human resource specialists need time to read about current legal changes and case law so that they can keep abreast of an organization's responsibilities in areas such as affirmative action, sexual harassment, and grounds for employee termination (Noe et al., 2008). Many analyses of role requirements will demand that managers invest monetary resources. These investments can include purchases of equipment such as computers, or the contracting of training programs to increase employees' knowledge and skills necessary for successful job performance.

Workplace Equity. Managers want to hire employees who believe in the value of an honest day's work. Productive employees believe that their efforts will lead to rewards, and that this link exists in the organizations where they currently work. They possess the necessary abilities to do their jobs well, and they are willing to constantly improve their skills given the demands of technological innovations and changing consumer preferences. Good employees also have the tools necessary to do their jobs well. Tools can include computers and cell phones, and they can also include advanced knowledge available through management-funded training programs. Clearly, managers are blessed if they have employees who have all of these desirable qualities. To continue their task of motivating these employees, managers now have to be concerned with workplace equity.

Equity refers to a balance between the resources employees give to an organization and the benefits they receive (Adams, 1965; Greenberg, 1990; 1997). Employees invest their knowledge, skills, time, energy, and other personal resources into their organization. They then receive benefits in the form of salaries, stock options, overtime pay, promotions, status-bringing titles, and perks such as corner offices and parking privileges. Employees calculate the resources they invest, and then try to develop an estimate of the benefits they should receive. They can do this by making comparisons with others in the community who have similar jobs. People argue to themselves that if they are auditors in an accounting firm and have brought in a certain number of clients, then they should be paid the same as other auditors with similar job accomplishments.

Sports fans are very familiar with these considerations of equity. Every year, there is media coverage of professional athletes who had very good years. They had contracts that called for an average salary at the beginning of the season, but they gained more yards, caught more passes, scored more touchdowns, or made more tackles than many others players with better contracts. So what do they do? They ask to be treated more equitably. They request that their contracts be renegotiated or, if they are free agents, seek higher salaries on the open market.

One of the most interesting aspects of the equity calculation process is that people compare themselves with alternatives that are consistent with lifestyles that they find reasonable (Thibaut & Kelley, 1959). If auditors prefer living in a medium-sized city in the Midwest, they do not make comparisons with colleagues in New York City or San Francisco. They make comparisons with auditors who live in cities of about the same size. Many people in mid-size communities are familiar with this comparison. In assessing the perceived equity of their salaries, they don't compare themselves with people holding down similar jobs in big cities such as New York or London. Even though they know that big city jobs may pay more, they don't want to live in one of them! They want to live in a smaller community, and so they compare themselves with others with similar ambitions.

If hardworking employees feel that the benefits they receive from the company are equitable, then they experience a sense of job satisfaction. As a result, they stay with their companies longer and can engage in organization-enhancing behaviors such as mentoring younger employees and joining professional associations where they can obtain cutting-edge skills (Adams, 1965; Allen et al., 2009). But the complex task of motivating workers is not yet complete. Employees always want more from their organizations, and managers need to know this fact.

Wanting More. At this point in the analysis of motivation, employees are working hard for their organizations. They will then examine whether or not they are being treated equitably. They will examine the rewards they receive, especially salaries, and will compare themselves with others who hold down similar jobs. If they feel the rewards they receive are comparable, they will feel equitably treated. If they feel inadequately rewarded, they will experience dissatisfaction and may leave their organizations.

If workers feel equitably treated, is the analysis of motivation complete? No, and the reason goes back to the early part of this discussion. Workers have various valences, and all must be satisfied. Further, even if they did not have a certain valence when they started working for a company, they might develop it over time. For example, people might take a job because they feel that it will satisfy their need to achieve and to receive recognition for their accomplishments. They may feel that they can satisfy this valence in their current organization and they may feel equitably treated. But they may find themselves becoming interested in supervising the work of others. Managing other people is quite different from the valences of achievement and recognition. Workers with this new valence will then examine whether or not their current job leads to positive outcomes and equity. If it does not, they will experience dissatisfaction. Does this mean that workers will never be entirely satisfied? The answer is yes. If people become satisfied with certain aspects of their lives, they will develop other needs that they want to fulfill (Porter & Lawler, 1968; Robinson, 2001). This is human nature, and it means that managers must always be attentive to the changing and increasing demands of their best workers.

READING SOCIAL SITUATIONS AS PART OF WORKER MOTIVATION

In analyzing worker motivation, managers must realize that people are different. They want different outcomes from their work, they have a variety of expectations, they have different abilities, and they have different feelings about equitable treatment. Managers can improve their own efforts to motivate workers if they keep in mind one of the themes discussed in several of this book's chapters: People react to the social situations in which they find themselves.

Social situations refer to influences on people's behavior that they experience in their day-to-day movements in their homes, workplaces, and community activities (Mischel, 2004; Zimbardo & Leippe, 1991; Zimbardo, 2007). Different elements in a social situation can have an influence on an individual's behavior, and these elements include other people. In a workplace with cubicles rather than offices, loud neighbors who talk with friends on their cell phones can be a major distraction. They contribute to quite a different social situation than considerate workplace neighbors who carefully monitor their voice levels.

There are several conceptualizations of behavior that give advice to managers and supervisors based on situational influences. The model developed by Paul Hersey and Kenneth Blanchard (1988) is based on all possible answers to two questions. Supervisors ask, "Do my employees have the ability to do the task that I want them to undertake?" And they ask, "Do my employees understand the importance of the task and are they motivated to putting out their best efforts?" The first question refers to employee ability and the second to their motivation and commitment. Managers have to read the situations in which workers find themselves and give themselves answers to the two questions. At times, employees can help by giving direct answers to the questions, but often they cannot and managers have to formulate answers with a minimum of verbal input from their employees.

If the answers to both questions are "no," then supervisors should engage in a leadership style that is both directive and supportive. This situation often arises with new hires. Supervisors need to oversee the training and mentoring of employees so that they acquire necessary skills. In addition, they need to support and to motivate the employees so that they will work hard, for the benefit of the company, after they acquire the necessary skills.

If employees have the necessary skills but lack commitment to the task that the supervisor wants completed, one-on-one coaching sessions are often effective (Allen et al., 2009). This situation often occurs with long-term employees who have lost some of their enthusiasm for their work. During the coaching sessions, supervisors can communicate their feelings about the importance of the task and their confidence that the employees can be successful if they put in the necessary time and effort.

If employees do not have the necessary skills but are highly motivated and committed, supervisors need to oversee programs that permit skill development (Martin, 1999). These can include on-the-job training, the encouragement of mentoring relationships, and off-site training where tuition is paid by the company. A key element is that employees are motivated to work hard. They need to be told what to do so that can combine their newly acquired job skills with their positive motivation.

If the answers to both questions are yes, indicating that employees are both skilled and committed, then supervisors can delegate (Hersey & Blanchard, 1988). They can tell the employees what outcomes are desired, for instance, specific production goals (Locke & Latham, 1984) or the development of a program for maintaining customer loyalty. Then, supervisors can let the employees develop their own plans for achieving the goals. With this type of employee, supervisors can then turn their attention to workplace issues demanding more of their own hands-on effort.

Using this model, supervisors adjust their behaviors and act differently toward their employees. In my experience, employees accept this differential treatment as long as supervisors communicate the reasons for their behavior (Bays, 2007; Brislin, 2008). Further, supervisors can explain that "as employees grow with the organization and demonstrate both competence and commitment, more work will be delegated. The successful completion of delegated tasks will lead to promotions."

My argument is that managers must learn to read the situations that their employees face and then intervene in different ways depending on the situation cues that they identify. Managers must resist the more common tendency to observe behaviors and to make conclusions that downplay situational influences (Miller & Ross, 1975; Zimbardo & Leippe, 1991; Brislin, 2008). Most often, individuals observe the behavior of others and make judgments about their personalities. People who don't talk to others at social gatherings are introverted. People who tell others what to do in the workplace are power hungry. People who don't contribute to charitable campaigns at work are cheap. But often, people's behavior is influenced by situational forces that are invisible to observers. Thinking about situational factors is time-consuming and difficult, but it leads to more accurate assessments of why people behave as they do (Blass, 2004; Zimbardo, 2007).

Let's look at each of the three examples of situational influence. People who don't talk to others at parties may not know anyone in attendance. If they were at social gatherings where they knew lots of attendees, they might be very talkative and animated. People who tell others what to do may be concerned about an impending deadline that, if not met, may mean lost business for a company. Individuals who do not contribute to charitable campaigns may have recently incurred financial obligations such as medical bills for an aging parent. Even though they have altruistic personalities and always try to help others, they may be so cash-strapped that they cannot contribute for several years.

Why are situational factors so rarely taken into account when we think about the behavior of other people? One reason is that we often do not know the situational pressures faced by others (Brislin, 2008;

Miller & Ross, 1975). And even if we wanted to know, questions posed to others about these factors may violate privacy norms. In a workplace, for instance, some people are willing to talk about their financial obligations to parents and some people are not. In contrast to their lack of knowledge about others, people know the situational pressures that they face. In their own lives, people know who is likely to be at the social gathering, what the deadline is for a proposal, and how much they can contribute to charities.

Another reason for inattention to situational forces is that people's socialization often places emphasis on context-free concepts such as the honesty, integrity, consistency of self, and personal responsibility. This is captured in Shakespeare's *Hamlet* when Polonius gives fatherly advice just before his son, Laertes, is to travel abroad: "This above all, to thine own self be true." Polonius did not tell his son to take into account situational factors when giving his rather vague and unhelpful advice about being true to oneself. Perhaps directors who take on the task of staging *Hamlet* recognize this unhelpfulness. Often, Polonius is presented as a windbag giving fatuous musings to a son who is clearly eager to escape a boring monologue.

Individuals can take advantage of the fact that they know their own situational pressures when they are tempted to make judgments about the behavior of others. They can make their observations and then ask, "In what sorts of situations would I act that way? What would make me be quiet at a party, act in a bossy manner, or come across as tight with my money?" Answers to such questions help individuals develop empathy (Miller & Rose, 2009), and this is an important contributor to their success in workplaces that attract the talents of people who have had very different life experiences.

SOME SUMMARY POINTS: WORKER MOTIVATION

A great deal of material has been covered in this chapter. Key points are summarized in Figure 11.1. The point of view presented in the figure is that of the manager who is responsible for the performance of motivated and productive employees.

Beginning at the upper-left corner of the figure (1), managers need to know what employees want from their work (Porter & Lawyer, 1968). Do they use want money (*Theory X*), or do they want their work to be part of positive self-identities (*Theory Y*, McGregor, 1960)? Managers should know the factors that protect employees from disliking their jobs (*hygienes*), as well as factors that contribute to feelings that people like their jobs (*motivators*, Herzberg et al., 1959).

With this knowledge, the next part of the figure (2) asks whether or not worker preferences are aligned with company goals. Managers should

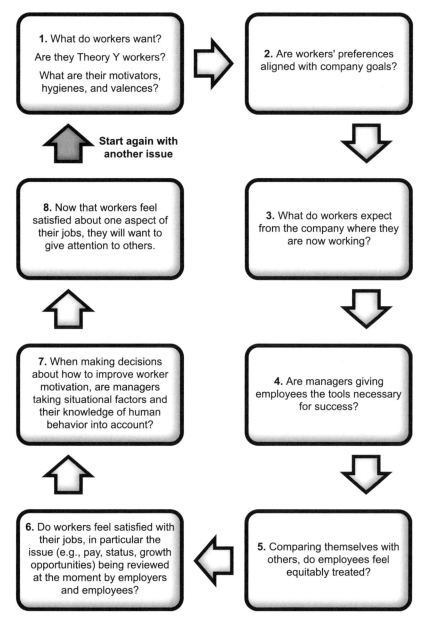

Figure 11.1 A Summary of Steps in Analyzing Worker Motivation.

know the motivational profiles of their employees and devise methods so that these profiles are linked to company goals. For example, employees who value creativity and innovation can be assigned tasks that could lead to new markets, products, or services for a company. Employees who value positive relations with others (often called the *affiliation motive*) can be asked to mentor new hires and to introduce the newcomers to colleagues in various departments within the organization (Allen et al., 2009).

Once managers become well acquainted with their employees, they are able to answer other questions (3). They should know what employees expect from their work. Do they want long-term employment, or do they plan to be with the company for no more than two or three years (De Cuyper et al., 2009)? Do they want to become active in professional organizations associated with the company? Have they labeled themselves as future executives and do they see opportunities to achieve this goal?

Employees need tools, broadly defined, to do their jobs (4). Tools can include items that can be touched, such as hammers, computers, and cell phones. But they can also include less physically clear career necessities such as introductions to influential networks (Brislin, 1991) and mentoring advice concerning intangible issues such as information concerning "the way things really work around here." In several organizations that I know, new hires with executive ambitions are expected to do voluntary work in the community that will reflect well on their organization. This expectation might not be written down in company policies, and so supervisors should be sure to explain the importance of voluntary work to their employees.

The next step in the analysis of motivation (5) is to assess whether or not workers feel equitably treated (Greenberg, 1990; 1997). This means that managers have to realize that workers compare themselves to peers. If peers with similar job qualifications, workplace contributions, and productivity are receiving certain wage-benefit packages, then workers want to be compensated equitably compared to these peers. The comparison group may not be all workers in all cities. If people from a medium-sized Midwestern city value their lifestyles there, then they will not compare themselves with age peers working in New York City or Los Angeles. Their comparison group will be workers from similar communities as the ones where they live.

At this point, workers have gone through steps 1 through 5 dealing with their preferences, alignment of their talents and expectations with their company and its goals, tools for success, and feelings of equity. Now, they decide if they are satisfied or not (step 6). Satisfied workers are likely to stay with the company rather than leave, contributing to company expenses if they are to be replaced. Satisfied workers are often good organizational citizens who make contributions above and beyond the tasks listed in their job descriptions (Farh et al., 2008).

Now, managers must add in what might be called *advanced knowledge* (step 7). They need to realize the importance of situational factors and must move away from the quick conclusion that worker traits cause all observed behaviors (Zimbardo, 2007). A tardy employee may not be lazy. There may be a sick child who needs care. Bewildered employees may not be uncaring. They may not have had sufficient experience with the task at hand to complete it successfully. Reading this situational cue, managers can intervene with coaching or referral to a training program.

Another piece of knowledge managers must have is the realization that workers will never be completely satisfied (Porter & Lawler, 1968; Robinson, 2001). If one aspect of their motivational profiles is satisfied, then they will want to pursue another (step 8). This means that they will start the motivational analysis again at step 1. If they are receiving satisfactory pay, they will give attention to perks such as parking and vacation time. If they feel that their creative needs are being met, they will seek to satisfy their affiliative needs or their desires for regular promotions. This never-ending quest for more is sometimes called *the revolution of rising expectations* (Robinson, 2001). Once people acquire some desired aspects that follow from their ambitions, they want more. They know the positive feeling that result from goal attainment, they see the possibility of more desirable outcomes coming their way, and they shift their attention to those additional outcomes.

12

Dealing with Prejudice and Embracing Diversity

Compared to 50 years ago, today's workplaces are much more diverse (Brislin, 2008; Noe et al., 2008). The typical employee of 50 years ago was an Anglo male; this is no longer the case. Today, there is much more workplace diversity, with more women, members of diverse ethnic and cultural groups, employees from different religious backgrounds, people with disabilities, people of diverse ages, and employees with different sexual orientations. Executives must deal effectively with such diversity if their companies are to thrive.

A common problem when members of these diverse groups interact is that one group may be favored at the expense of another (Allport, 1954; Brewer, 2007). In this chapter, research on negative feelings toward outgroups will be analyzed, and research on overcoming hostile ingroup-outgroup relations will be reviewed.

PREJUDICE

Whenever people from different cultural backgrounds come together, there is the danger of reactions that are based on prejudice (Allport, 1954; Pettigrew, 1998). This term *prejudice* is complex and has many aspects, but a good start at understanding it is to look at the root terms. *Pre* means before, and here it refers to people's reactions that occur before first-hand experiences and before careful thought. The second part of the term refers to *judging*. People, when confronted with differences, make judgments based on those observed differences and avoid the hard work necessary to understand specific people. There are various forms that prejudice takes, and each deserves discussion for its workplace implications.

Forms of Prejudice: Racism. The best known, and most difficult form to change, is old-fashioned racism. If people have prejudiced views that are racist, they believe that other groups of people have less ability, are less intelligent, and should take jobs that don't demand much more than unskilled labor. Often, racism is learned during childhood and young people are taught not to associate with members of certain other groups because it will bring shame to their families (Allport, 1954). Racist beliefs are often aimed at people from other cultural groups whose members have different skin colors, languages, and everyday means of satisfying life's basic requirements.

Racism has the terribly unfortunate set of beliefs that people in other groups are inferior by the very fact of their birth or biology. Thus people guilty of racism believe that the targets of their prejudices just can't help themselves. "They were born that way and so it's a waste of time to try to do much about it." Such beliefs put the others at a disadvantage. If they are considered inferior, they are not chosen to be interviewed for career-developing positions and instead become shunted aside into dead-end jobs.

Other intense prejudices are similar to racism in that they deal with birth or a biological fact about people (Aosved, Long, & Voller, 2009). These prejudice are sometimes referred to as the "isms" and deal with gender-based groups (sexism), the physically disabled, older people (ageism), or people who are not physically attractive (lookism). The similarity to racism is that people, because of a biological fact, are given a label that has major implications for their chances at finding happiness. They are denied societal benefits that are available only to those with the power to put their racist beliefs into the maintenance of discriminatory social policies (Brislin, 2000).

Prejudices based on racism are extremely difficult to change (Amir, 1969; Pettigrew, 1998). Many of these prejudices stem from people's childhood years, the time they were learning what society considers right and wrong. Unfortunately, many people learn that it is "right" to treat others as if they are inferior. Sometimes, years and years of positive experiences with members of other groups help people overcome the prejudices of their childhood. At other times, people approach prejudice reduction through their religious beliefs. A person from Texas once told me, "I grew up with a prejudice against African Americans. Studying the Bible, I came to the conclusion that this was simply not right. I now run a business and hire people from all the local ethnic groups. And I pray every day that I can behave in a decent way toward everyone."

Tokenism. Educational television stations frequently offer concerts by symphony orchestras, and I enjoy watching them. Camera shots offer views of the entire orchestra and also close-ups of individual musicians. During one program, one of the best-known American orchestras offered a program of Beethoven, Mozart, and Prokofiev. There were more than 100 people playing, and I noticed exactly one African American musician seated deep in the strings section. I remember saying, "This is an example of tokenism that I'll have to remember when I talk to groups about prejudice and intergroup relations."

When people are prejudiced, they harbor negative attitudes about people from other groups with different traits such as skin color, nationality, and accent within their language. People express their prejudiced attitudes in different ways. Some people are very direct in their expression. They openly tell friends and colleagues that they don't like members of certain outgroups, feel that they are inferior, and that their country would be better off without them (Cingoz-Ulu & Lalonde, 2007). Other people are much more indirect in their expression. Often well-educated, these people know that there are social norms and legal repercussions that discourage open expression of intense prejudices. Given this awareness, these more indirect people sometimes engage in token behaviors toward members of other groups.

Although positive in nature, these token behaviors offer minimum benefits to outgroup members. The symphony orchestra that I saw on television has engaged in a token behavior by hiring one African American. Orchestra executives can point to the one violinist as evidence of a policy of encouraging minority employees. With this token gesture (Wright & Taylor, 1999), the executives can continue to avoid more vigorous actions that would create a more positive atmosphere of intergroup tolerance.

In different organizations, token behaviors can take place at various stages of people's career development. Many people from minority groups may be offered job interviews, but only a few may be hired. Once on the job, these few minority group members may find that only one or two are offered advanced training programs that can lead to promotions and salary increases. Or, just one or two may be offered membership in local clubs where managers and executives from various organizations develop the networks necessary for career advancement (Thomas et al., 1996).

Executives can engage in other types of token behaviors. Members of minority groups may want to meet regularly to discuss issues in their organizations. They may want to formulate recommendations about minority issues that they will present to senior-level managers. Executives might encourage this and offer the use of the most prestigious meeting rooms. The executives may even prepare a press release about the meetings and send it to newspapers and television stations. These executive behaviors may be meaningless tokens. Minority group members may feel well treated, but there is no guarantee that there will be any action. In some parts of the world, executives may know that the minority group members will probably squabble among themselves and fail to reach agreement concerning recommendations (Brislin, 1991). But the executives can say, "We gave them every opportunity!"

Likes and Dislikes. People have features that are visible to others with whom they come into contact. Many times, these differences can lead to conclusions that "some people are like me and so are part of my group, and others are different and so should be thought of as members of another group." Differences can be based on physical features such as gender, skin color, age, disabilities, and choices of clothing. Differences can also be based on behaviors such as how often people speak up in public gatherings and whether or not they take disagreements personally when discussing important issues in an organization (Fassinger, 2008).

When people from one group interact with people from another, there is always the possibility of misunderstandings and negative reactions (Barna, 2009; Hyun, 2005). Many times, these reactions are based on real likes and dislikes. People develop preferred ways of behaving over their lifetimes, and they decide that other ways of behaving are unacceptable, inefficient, or rude. But as part of their everyday intergroup relations, people may interact with others for whom these other unpreferred behaviors are quite acceptable. For example, most well-educated American adults do not have a smoking habit. Less than 20 percent of American middle-class adults smoke, and this is an extremely large difference when considering behaviors that lead people to form groups (e.g., people who behave like I do compared to others).

But if Americans travel to Asian countries, they will interact with many smokers and will eat in restaurants where second-hand smoke fills the air. Many Asian countries have not enacted laws that provide for smoke-free restaurants, bars, and enclosed office spaces. This difference between Americans and Asians, based on a real dislike, can have an impact on decisions regarding personal and business travel.

Behaviors common in the workplace often lead to the feeling that there is more than one group present (Brislin, 2008; Thomas et al., 1996). Many recent arrivals from the mainland United States were socialized to speak up in public meetings, to voice their complaints openly, and to disagree with others in the pursuit of better decisions within their organizations. Many locals in Hawaii were socialized to be careful about speaking up in public. They were taught that it is better to seek consensus through quiet negotiation rather than through open disagreement and confrontation. Mainlanders are surprised to find that they have been labeled as loudmouths in the workplace. I recently attended a meeting in Hawaii where the job description for a high-ranking executive position was being discussed. People at the meeting agreed that the executive could be ambitious, have lofty goals, and move the organization toward major changes; however, he or she would have to do this in a quiet, nonconfrontational manner that does not cause others to lose face.

People often have to make decisions based on behaviors that they like and dislike. People decide to pursue relationships with others for many reasons, and the presence or absence of a smoking habit has an impact. In the Hawaiian workplace example, many people from the mainland must decide if they can put aside their preferred direct and confrontational style in favor of a softer, harmony-seeking approach to decision making. If they cannot, they may find themselves on an airplane back to the mainland.

Unfamiliar Behaviors. Whenever a large number of people come together, they are likely to form group ties based on shared physical characteristics, behaviors, or interests. People in one's ingroup share perceived similarities. People have positive feelings about members of their ingroups and enjoy interacting with them. Individuals in one's outgroup are different in some way. They look different, have a language or accent that can't be understood, or behave in ways considered unacceptable to the person making judgments about group membership.

The formation of ingroups and outgroups is universal and is a basic fact that marks human beings, similar to the needs for food, water, and sleep (Brewer, 2007). Many people make decisions about their behavior based on their ingroups and outgroups. For example, we might consider all candidates running for elective office and vote for those who will best represent all the people in Hawaii. But we don't. Instead, we divide candidates into ingroups and outgroups. In many parts of the world, the ethnic vote (my group and other groups) is a factor that politicians must consider if they are to be elected. When executives favor candidates from certain ethnic groups for jobs in their organizations, they are behaving according to ingroup and outgroup distinctions. Such choices are sometimes unconscious. The executives simply prefer candidates who share similarities and who seem familiar (Kahneman & Tversky, 2000).

The danger of ingroup and outgroup formation is that others considered different are sometimes put at a disadvantage in their quest for society's benefits. Often, especially with people who are trying to be sensitive to others and to put racist feelings aside, ingroup and outgroup distinctions are based on what is familiar and unfamiliar to people (Brislin, 2000). These distinctions are especially prominent when people move from one city to another and must learn new behaviors that will allow them to satisfy everyday needs. People moving from the mainland United States to Hawaii face the need to engage in many unfamiliar behaviors. Examples are attending baby luaus, learning new terms such as *pau* (it's finished or completed), *hapa* (half), and *niele* (nosy, overly intrusive with one's curiosity), and making sure that others do not lose face during interpersonal interactions.

The inclusion of the familiar and unfamiliar in discussions about prejudice may seem out of place. Prejudices based on racist beliefs seem far removed from ingroup-outgroup misunderstandings based on unfamiliar behaviors. I include them in the same discussion because the outcomes are similar. People from different groups do not interact frequently or smoothly. They are not benefiting from the stimulation provided when diverse people interact, share their varied perspectives, and arrive at decisions that are better because people have integrated complex viewpoints (Thomas et al., 1996).

Ingroup and outgroup misunderstandings based on unfamiliar behaviors are relatively easy to address. In a diverse workplace, for example, executives can ask the question, "What are differences that, over the years, have caused misunderstandings among people here in the workplace?" In a large organization, human resource specialists can be brought in to add to the list of differences. Then, these differences can be explained to everyone as part of formal training programs, mentoring activities in the workplace, and during informal conversations (Singelis, 1998).

If people are not familiar with other groups or other parts of the world, they often make decisions based on oversimplifications (Khan & Liu, 2008) that they have learned from the media or from conversations with others who have had equally scanty direct experiences. This is an issue in this incident.

Views of People from Other Groups Are Often Oversimplified

"This is a tempting offer," Janice Ozawa told a colleague at work. Janice, who had spent most of her life in Honolulu, was recently offered a job in the home office of the financial institution where she worked. The home office was in New York City, a place Janice had visited twice on vacations. She faced a classic dilemma that many people in Hawaii experience. The salary for the New York job was higher, but she was concerned that she would miss her family in Hawaii. Further, she loved Hawaii's climate and lifestyle.

Sharing her concerns with her colleague, she voiced another concern. "All the people in New York seem so rushed and are always in a hurry to do something. I've never been shoved around so much as when I was walking on busy streets in New York!" Her colleague responded, "Try not to oversimplify. Not everyone in New York is as you describe."

Janice is guilty of what is known as the outgroup homogeneity effect (Denhaerinck, Leyens, & Yzerbyt, 1989). Outgroups refer to people whom we do not know very well and with whom we do not have day-to-day contact. When thinking about outgroups, there is a tendency to conclude that members are pretty much the same. This is especially true if we know just a few things about outgroup members, as in Janice's limited contact with New Yorkers during her vacations. So if she had experiences with fast-moving and rude outgroup members, she may conclude that everyone in New York behaves the same way.

This perceptual error stands in interesting contrast to the way we think about people whom we know well. In the ingroup heterogeneity effect, we recognize differences among people (Triandis, 1995; 2009). The term *ingroups* refers to individuals who are close to us, who share their emotional ups and downs, and who we look forward to seeing. We recognize the differences, or the heterogeneity, among these people. Some are always in a rush and some are laid back. Some always arrive at the advertised starting time for weekend company picnics, and some show up a few hours late. Some like to travel to Las Vegas to gamble and some prefer to travel to music festivals. We recognize these differences because we are very familiar with ingroup members.

A good way to become more aware of the outgroup homogeneity effect is to put ourselves in the shoes of outsiders. Consider people from New York thinking about residents of Hawaii. They are likely to imagine that everyone in Hawaii loves surfing, spends weekends at the beach, belongs to a hula group, and plays the ukulele. Residents of Hawaii know that this is a terrible oversimplification. But if we realize this, we can entertain the possibility that our views of people in other parts of the world are likely to downplay the vast differences among individuals.

The outgroup homogeneity effect can lead to odd complications. People on the mainland not only feel that Hawaii residents are similar, but that we all constantly talk to each other! Like many residents, I receive letters and e-mails from mainlanders who want jobs. They send their resumes, thinking that Hawaii residents know dozens of executives who are on the hiring committees for high-paying jobs in banking, real estate, and the tourist industry. If they thought about their own communities that they know well, the job seekers would realize that not everyone has close relations with executives in all types of businesses.

OVERCOMING PREJUDICE

Prejudices can be changed and companies can become more egalitarian (Cohen & Insko, 2008). Organizations can develop a reputation as being good places to work regardless of people's ethnicity, religion, gender, or other reason that might lead to the formation of ingroups and outgroups. But achieving this goal takes a great deal of time, effort, and investment of resources. In this section, I will present recommendations based on research studies that have dealt with the goal of prejudice reduction.

Administrative Support. The first requirement is that a company's executives must vigorously support programs aimed at prejudice reduction and improved intergroup relations (Ely & Thomas, 2001; Lim & Guo, 2008). Administrators must make it clear that an organization's employees cannot engage in discriminatory behavior and cannot show evidence of negative attitudes toward any group of people. Executives must demonstrate this type of tolerance in their own behavior (Aronson and Patnoe, 1997; Brislin, 2000). In other words, executives must become models of the behaviors that they want employees to emulate. Over a period of years, employees become very skillful at making distinctions between what executives say and what the executives actually want. If executives pay only "lip service" to improved intergroup relations, then employees will not change their behaviors. Executives must make their goals clear, and they must communicate to employees that there will be consequences if the goals are not met.

Equal Status. Another requirement is that all employees have equal status within the organization regardless of their group memberships (ethnicity, gender, perceived disability, and so forth). This requirement follows from the analysis of administrative support since a company's executives have to oversee and enforce efforts to achieve equal status. The goal of equal status means that everyone in the organization has equal access to rewards and benefits (Aronson & Patnoe, 1997; Boldry & Gaertner, 2006). These include outcomes such as jobs with the highest salaries, paid attendance at training programs to improve job skills, and invitations to meetings where company policy is set.

Many times, administrators will have to pursue goals for positive intergroup relations that do not exist in the larger society. They will have to say, "There may be prejudice and discrimination in different parts of this city. People from minority groups may not have access to the best schools, membership in prestigious social clubs, and other opportunities to improve themselves. However, in this organization this type of prejudice and discrimination will not be tolerated. Everyone will have equal access to all benefits that employment in this company can offer." In addition to their verbal communications, executives will advance their goals if they identify and reward employees whose behavior clearly indicates that they accept these policies.

Superordinate Goals. People are very sensitive to features that make one individual different from another. At times, individuals emphasize these features and want to have the reputation of being different from others on selected dimensions. These features leading to judgments about and emphases of differences include skin color, age, gender, social class, and section of a country where a person grew up. Many times, these differences lead to judgments concerning various evaluations. Who is smarter? Who is better looking? Who is a better leader? Who is more dependable in the workplace? Who is better prepared to interact with the company's most important customers? People who feel that they are similar often form groups, spend time with each other, and exchange favors. When behaving in this way, they exclude individuals who are seen as different.

The feelings generated by attention to these differences often work against the goals of a company. If energy is spent on forming and maintaining ingroup alliances and outgroup derision, then energy is drained away from company goals such as product development and good customer service (Thomas et al., 1996; Thomas & Inkson, 2009). If executives want to improve a company's intergroup relations, there are various steps that they can take. One of the most important is that executives, after consulting with employees, should formulate goals that everyone in the workplace accepts as important.

These desired organizational outcomes, called *superordinate goals* (Sherif, 1966) demand both the acceptance and efforts of all employees. Superordinate goals cannot be achieved by one or a few people: the efforts of all are clearly needed (Pettigrew, 1998; 2008). Executives need to ensure that everyone sees the importance of these goals and understands how their contributions are needed. If this can be done, petty backbiting and irrelevant ingroup-outgroup squabbles will take a distant second place to the positive energies of common group effort. My father captured this in advice to his children. The family moved several times during our challenging teenage years, and so we were faced with the task of developing new friendships. My father advised, "Join clubs that seem important to people at the school. By working with people on shared activities, you'll help the club and also make friends. You will quickly move from being an outsider to a club member."

It is useful to identify places where the results of effective intergroup relations can be seen. Let's consider a college campus. Where are positive intergroup relations essential? One place is the athletic department. Men and women from very different backgrounds come together and must work together toward group goals. Differences can be due to race, ethnicity, religion, the local-nonlocal distinction common in Hawaii, and the status and wealth of parents. However, these distinctions have to be set aside if members of an athletic team are to work toward goals such as a winning season and participation in postseason tournaments. People from different backgrounds do not have to become close friends, although they often do. They must set aside differences that have no bearing on team performance and work together toward shared team goals. If they put energy into maintaining irrelevant ingroup-outgroup distinctions, there will be a place for them on the bench rather than on the court or playing field.

Breaking Stereotypes. Another managerial intervention likely to lead to improvements is that contact among people should break existing stereotypes (Baretto, Ryan, & Schmitt, 2009). Whenever people from different groups come together and interact, there are always generalizations about the groups that ignore individual differences and that may be very unfair. The unfairness is due to the imposition of perceived limits. If people are stereotyped, they may not be given opportunities in areas beyond the limits of the stereotype. For example, if there is the stereotype that women are not good at tasks involving complex mathematics, a highly skilled woman may be overlooked when executives assign tasks to employees. Generalizations about people or stereotypes are too often used in organizational decision making and in people's decisions concerning whom they will interact with in an organization (Adler, 2002).

Executives can combat the impact of stereotypes by making sure that facile generalizations about groups of people are challenged. At company meetings, for example, they can ask people to make different kinds of contributions. If the stereotype exists that locals in Hawaii are slow to speak up in meetings, executives can ask locals to present a set of recommendations for company action. If recent arrivals from the mainland United States have the reputation for telling people in Hawaii what they should do, executives can ask the mainlanders to facilitate a group discussion where everyone is expected to contribute. If a certain group has the reputation of producing good athletes, individuals can be asked to make contributions that demand high-level conceptual skills relevant to the organization's mission.

One reason why stereotype-breaking contact is effective is that it provides challenges to people's thinking (Kahneman & Tversky, 2000). Everyone is extremely busy with day-to-day activities in their workplaces, homes, churches, and community activities. People do not have time to think carefully about all decisions they face and instead rely on shortcuts such as stereotypes. But when people break a stereotypical label through their actions and contributions, this forces others to think about what has happened. They are encouraged to move beyond their everyday casual thinking and to consider reasons for the unexpected behaviors they have observed. Since they have put mental energy into these considerations, they are likely to remember the exceptions to the stereotypes. Over time, people will hopefully see so many exceptions that the original stereotypes are discarded.

Creating More Inclusive Social Identities. When people are asked to describe themselves, they demonstrate that their identities are complex. All people have a sense of the individual self and can describe themselves with adjectives: "I am talkative, I am aggressive when negotiating, I am dependable," and so forth. People also have a sense of the collective self (Tajfel, 1981) and can describe themselves in terms of group memberships and relations with other people: "I am a parent, I am a member of a paddling club, I am a graduate of Roosevelt High School," and so forth. These various aspects of people's identities can be very flexible. Talkative people, for example, might practice with their paddling clubs in the afternoon and attend a high school alumni meeting in the evening. Their behaviors will be guided both by their individual traits and the group memberships that are prominent at any one time. People can adapt their traits according to their group memberships. Talkative people, for example, might listen respectfully when more experienced paddlers give instructions and as they catch up with old friends at the high school alumni meeting.

Many times, the collective aspects of people's identities can be so strong that other individuals are labeled as members of outgroups because reasons for a shared identity cannot be readily identified (Brewer, 2007). The clearest examples occur when people consider their ethnic group membership as a major part of their identities. If people claim Filipino American as their only ethic affiliation, then they can't be Japanese Americans or Irish Americans. Strong ethnic affiliations can lead to discrimination against others (Tajfel, 1981). If businesspeople from one ethnic group favor people who share this affiliation in decisions such as hirings and promotions, then outgroup members are put at a disadvantage.

This can lead to a major problem for organizations. If people are hired and promoted because of group memberships rather than potential contributions to the workplace, then the organization will suffer because it is not making the best use of its talent. Executives should consider this as a problem that demands their intervention efforts.

Executives can take the forward-looking step of benefitting from people's flexible social identities (Tajfel, 1981; Triandis, 1995). Just as they can be both members of a canoe club and loyal alumni of a high school, people can have multiple identities that will bring benefits to their workplaces. If executives are able to increase organizational morale, for example, people will shift their identities from "wage employee" to "proud employee" of a specific organization. They can retain their strong ethnic group affiliation, but they can also develop the identity as people who work in an organization where the talents of many ethnic groups are welcome and encouraged. People thus develop multiple and overlapping group ties (Pettigrew, 1998; 2008). One tie, such as ethnic identity, is not weakened because people have the additional identity of employment in a company of which they are proud.

Dealing in a Candid Manner with Difficulties. Improving intergroup relations is difficult and potential problems must be openly addressed and discussed. No benefits will accrue if executives sweep problems under the rug and pretend that they don't exist (Dixon, Durrheim, & Tredoux, 2005). One potential difficulty is that employees have multiple roles. They work for an organization and are also neighbors in a community and members of various voluntary associations. Employees may come to recognize the benefits of positive intergroup relations in the workplace. However, they may drive home to communities where neighbors maintain sharp ingroup and outgroup ties with the help of gender-, ethnic-, and class-based epithets. This is the sort of problem that should be openly discussed at workplace meetings. Employees may decide to learn social skills that allow them to contribute to company goals and to maintain good standing in their neighborhoods. These skills include learning how to say "no" politely, changing the subject of neighborhood conversations, and challenging the negative feelings behind the epithets in a nonthreatening manner.

Another problem can occur if the desired outcomes of improved intergroup relations are too overblown (Dixon et al., 2005). Goals should be realistic, such as respect in the workplace regardless of group ties and equal access to promotions and advanced training programs. People from different groups may not necessarily become best friends. If this becomes a company goal, executives may become discouraged when employees do not start socializing with each other during evenings and on weekends. Adults interact based on shared interests, and many times these interests were developed during childhood. Whether it is grand opera, line dancing, cricket, arguing politics, or bluegrass music, people from one group may find the activity interesting while others find it an unattractive use of their time. Perhaps people will eventually expand their interests and will interact more outside the workplace, but executives should not establish such interaction as a short-term goal. If they focus on equal opportunities and benefits in the workplace (Sherif, 1966), executives will make a major contribution to improved intergroup relations and to the reduction of prejudice.

SOME COMPLEXITIES IN THE ANALYSIS OF PREJUDICE

Now that the nature of prejudice has been analyzed, as well as ways of overcoming it, I would now like to analyze some examples that involve various kinds of complexities. The three examples involve social class, insensitivities to the viewpoints of others, and the possibility of places in the world with less prejudice than others.

Social Class. Most of the discussion of prejudice in this chapter has involved interactions among people from different ethnic groups. Prejudice can involve interactions among people from many different types of backgrounds, including social class (Aosved et al., 2009).

People's behavior is determined by multiple causes. This very important statement is at odds with the common thought that behaviors and causes line up in one-to-one relationships. For example, people who don't volunteer for community development activities are seen as selfish. People who cut in and out of traffic are reckless. In several chapters, including this one, I have discussed the importance of a more complex view of human behavior. I have emphasized personality-situation combinations that better explain behavior. In the case of volunteer activities, some people will become very active if asked to do so. They won't raise their hand when a work committee is called for, but they will be diligent with their time and effort if asked to participate. People who drive in an unsafe manner may be rushing a family member to the hospital because of a medical emergency.

Other reasons for people's behavior stem from their life experiences (Snibbe & Markus, 2005). If people have dealt with social situations in the same way for many years, they are likely to continue these behaviors when faced with similar situations today. Some of these behaviors stem from people's social class background, also frequently called their socioeconomic status. Social class is often measured by four criteria: the amount of education people have received, their income, the neighborhood in which they live, and subjective ratings of people's occupations. The criteria are often interrelated. If people have many years of formal education, they often obtain good-paying and prestigious jobs. Given their incomes, they can afford to live in more expensive neighborhoods.

A knowledge of social class background helps in thinking about workplace behavior. When counseling people about job problems, many complaints focus on unreasonable customers. Workers complain that customers are rude, make unreasonable demands, and use foul language. The workers often try to guess the ethnic background of these impolite customers based on physical features. Then, they want to conclude that such behavior is widespread in certain groups. I urge the workers not to make conclusions based on ethnicity. Instead, the behavior may be due to social class background, and the different socio-economic levels are present in every ethnic group (Bernstein, 1971).

I will make some generalizations about social class, and there are certainly exceptions. If people were born into or have achieved middle- and higher-level socioeconomic levels, they have been exposed to inter-personal skills that are more effective than shouting and cursing. If workers are addressed in a soft and respectful way, they are more likely to invest their time and energy into satisfying customer requests. Such gentle social skills stem from the criteria of social class. People with a college education have met many different kinds of individuals and have learned to get along with them. This is especially true if some of their college friends and acquaintances are from other countries (Thomas & Inkson, 2009). If they are to receive promotions and corre-sponding salary increases in their chosen professions, they must dem-onstrate gentle social skills and must interact with others in a cooperative and respectful manner. Given their income, they can then afford to live in neighborhoods where a pleasant communication style is the norm. In these neighborhoods, people are constantly exposed to communication styles that mark individuals who are known as "classy" and as socially skilled.

Aspects of employees' backgrounds, as in this discussion of social class, can affect their behavior in the workplace.

Subtle Behaviors That May Escape Discussion. At times, managers will make every attempt to interact with employees in a fair, unbiased, and unprejudiced manner. However, their attempts may still be taken as signs of discrimination (Simons, Friedman, Liu, & McLean-Parks, 2007), as in this incident.

Worker Sensitivities May Lead to Charges of Prejudice

Given his own background from a working-class family whose father escaped Hungary during the 1956 revolution, Walt Sommers tried to be sensitive to others in his role as manager of an auto supply company. The last three years at his company had been good, with increasing sales and year-end bonuses to all employees. Walt decided to introduce an incentive plan. The three workers with the largest sales volume would receive funds to attend a leadership development program in a city where many company employees choose to spend their vacations. Participation in the leadership program was seen as a desirable feature in applications for promotion within the company.

At the end of the competition, three workers knew that their sales were the highest in the company. One of them was Valerie Baxter, an African American, and the other two were Anglo males. Unfortunately, Walt had to announce that the incentive program, and its award of the trip, had to be cancelled. The company had just gone through a bad year given a general economic recession in the entire country. The two Anglos shrugged their shoulders and went back to work. They had reactions such as, "I know that the company has been going through tough economic times," and, "Maybe they will take our sales performance into account when the economy turns around, allowing them to offer incentives again." Valerie, on the other hand, felt that Walt had not followed through on his promises. "I'll never be able to trust him again," she said to herself.

Recent research has shown that members of minority groups are often more sensitive to workplace episodes in which trust may be involved (Simons et al., 2007). Minorities are more likely to observe managerial behavior, and if they disapprove of the behavior, are more likely to formulate negative attributions. "Again, we are getting the short end of the stick," is one possible verbalization among others that are more colorful. One reason is that minorities are more likely to have experienced prejudice and discrimination in the past. They then can interpret current difficulties as just one more example of how minorities are not allowed access to the same societal benefits as members of the dominant Anglo group.

Another reason is that members of minority groups, growing up in their societies, had to be attentive toward majority members so as to figure out how majority people behave and how to obtain goals in the majority-dominated power structure. There is much more activity involving observation of majority members by minority members than observational activities in the other direction. This means that minority members, such as Valerie, will be more practiced in observing powerful members of the Anglo majority. As she observes Walt making the announcement concerning the abandonment of the incentive program, she is more likely to be attentive to his body language, his voice tone, his attempts at humor, and his explanation for the change. If she feels that something is amiss in any of Walt's verbal or nonverbal behaviors, she is likely to make the conclusion that Walt is not sincere and is not to be trusted in the future.

It is hard for me to give advice to Walt and to Valerie that will lead to a perfect or near-perfect solution to their problem. About all I could do would be to explain the issue of greater minority sensitivity to Walt, and to caution Valerie about making personal attributions about Walt that are situationally influenced (the unfavorable economy). People who pride themselves on positive intergroup relations in their workplaces must constantly give attention to this goal. The goal is not one that can seemingly be achieved and then taken for granted. Constant attention, and the realization that difficulties will always arise, is necessary.

The Case of Hawaii. In this chapter, I have discussed potential difficulties that can occur when people from very different cultural backgrounds interact frequently. I discussed the problems associated with prejudice, such as denying benefits to people because of group memberships based on factors such as ethnicity, gender, age, or social class. I also discussed ways of overcoming prejudice in organizations, such as strong executive direction, the development of shared goals, activities that move beyond group stereotypes, and the formation of new group identities that emphasize positive intergroup relationships.

Given that I have lived in the state for over 35 years, people often ask me whether I think that intergroup relations in Hawaii are better or worse than in other states and in other countries. My opinion is that although Hawaii is not a paradise in terms of group tolerance and there are ways to improve (Howard, 1964; Okamura, 2008), relations here are much more positive than in many other parts of the world. There are people in Hawaii who disagree, and so I will give reasons for my position.

Differing positions on important social issues often start with people's expectations. Many people expect intergroup relations to be favorable because they have heard or read about Hawaii's positive reputation as a model of tolerance. Then, when people observe a number of spats, conflicts, and unpleasant interactions that bedevil individuals everywhere, they may conclude that Hawaii is no better than anyplace else. My own starting point is different. I believe that it is difficult and challenging for people to interact when they do not share a common cultural background.

A common background provides many bases for smooth interactions: shared interests, similar meanings given to nonverbal behaviors, respect for certain authority figures who have a right to intervene in conflicts, and socially approved ways of disagreeing with others. When people from different cultural backgrounds come together, they do not share these bases for smooth conversations, interpretations of potentially problematic behaviors, and methods for smoothing over misunderstandings. People must invest extra time and effort into their interactions with culturally different individuals, and this can lead to extra burdens in lives already busy with work, family, and community activities (Barna, 2009).

Newcomers who decide to live in Hawaii must be willing to take on the extra task of learning enough about cultural differences so that they can have smooth interactions with others. If they decide that this is too burdensome, then they often get on an airplane and go elsewhere. As a result, there is a selection effect. People willing to purse the goal of positive intercultural relations stay in Hawaii, and others leave. These people also learn that there are many benefits to positive relations. Businesses in Hawaii have to cater to a small population, and employees cannot alienate potential customers from any one cultural group. Life in neighborhoods is much more pleasant if people can show respect for others in their day-to-day interactions. If they live in Hawaii long enough, people often develop kin relations with other cultural groups because of their children's marriages. By this time, they know that if they have difficulties with other cultures, then they have to live with the stress of poor relations with nearby relatives. People often come to the conclusion, then, that if they are to live in a multicultural society they will find much more success and happiness if they make attempts to make contributions toward smooth intercultural relations.

13

Personal and Organizational Change

Whenever people review a list of topics that have been covered in this book, they frequently come to the conclusion, "I have to make some changes, my organization needs to change, or both!" For example, people might admit that they need to improve their social skills or become more sophisticated about political influences in their workplaces. Or, they may decide that they should take advantage of the research on decision making and learn to make distinctions between decisions whose formulations do and do not need large amounts of time, effort, and energy. In thinking about their organization, executives may decide that to keep up with the competition, workers must become more motivated and productivity oriented. Or, executives may recognize their own mortality and conclude that there should be some leadership development programs to assist with a smooth transition after they leave the scene. In all these cases, people need to know about the difficulties surrounding change attempts as well as steps they can take to ease the difficulties (Carnall, 1990; Furnham, 2002; Marquardt, Leonard, Freedman, & Hill, 2009).

Change is difficult (D'Aprix, 2009). This is not the conclusion that people might make after hearing presentations by motivational speakers who might pop in and pop out of an organization. Motivational speakers are frequently invited into organizations and to conferences sponsored by various professional societies and membership organizations. Speakers are expected to fire up their listeners and to make them more enthusiastic about meeting their personal and organizational goals. The same motivational speakers can speak to groups about the importance of increasing the number of sales calls, accepting new technologies, improving customer service, and opening new niche markets. Speakers are often very exciting people who have the presentation skills of professional entertainers. Listeners often leave presentations with seemingly endless energy and the conviction that they can change themselves and their organizations. Just as often, their success resembles the changes brought on after their most recent set of New Year's resolutions.

INDIVIDUAL CHANGE

In this chapter, both personal and organizational change will be discussed, and I will start with modifications that people want to make in their own everyday behaviors. Change in long-established personal behaviors is very difficult and time-consuming. One reason, too infrequently discussed, is that people reap benefits from current behaviors they claim they want to change. Bosses who admit that they are crabby with subordinates get a pleasurable emotional surge when they exercise their ability to belittle and to raise their voices. Smokers who say they want to quit are comfortable having something to do with their hands during social encounters where they would otherwise be ill at ease. Shy people who want to become friendlier with others have an excuse for not going to social events where they might improve their business networks (Zimbardo, 1977; Zimbardo & Leippe, 1991). "I'm shy, and so I would not enjoy the social gathering where I know so few other people!"

Change demands the unfreezing of old behaviors, movement toward new desired goals, and enough practice and everyday experience to form new habits. This series of steps takes effort (Sherif, Sherif, & Nebergall, 1965). In the three examples, nicotine from the smoking habit is addictive, but so are the other old behaviors. Bosses get pleasure from shouting at others since it allows them to exercise their need for power. Shy people become addicted to their habit of turning down social invitations since it keeps them from the perceived unpleasantness of meeting and interacting with strangers. People have to put a great deal of conscious effort into imagining themselves after the change, and then regulating and monitoring their everyday behaviors so that they become consistent with their new goals (Baumeister & Vohs, 2007).

The self-regulation needed to think about and modify one's behaviors is energy draining. Many people cannot regulate more than one behavior at a time. If people are making attempts to cut down on their drinking, they have to monitor their intake, think about what social invitations to accept, and stay away from tempting places such as liquor departments in grocery stores. Given all the other demands on their lives due to their families, jobs, and community activities, most people find that there are limits to their self-regulation time and energy. If they try to change a second behavior, such as to show more enthusiasm about technical innovations in the workplace, they may experience the frustration of finding that their self-regulation limitations have been exceeded (Baumeister & Vohs, 2007).

ORGANIZATIONAL CHANGE

Readers might now say, "You discussed individual change and gave examples such as the behavior of a boss who wants to improve communication with subordinates or how people might work on changing a bad habit. In the place I work, I would like to see major changes throughout the organization that would affect everyone. If personal change is hard, is there any hope for changing my organization?"

Organizational changes demand the efforts of many people (Carnall, 1990; Gladwell, 2000; Van Iddekinge et al., 2009). The rantings and ravings of just one person are likely to go unnoticed. Any one person has to forge collaborative ties with others who may be thinking that the same proposed change would be desirable (Crick, 1982). Assume two individuals have lunch together and decide that they would like to see more involvement of company members in various community organizations. They feel that the company and the community would benefit from employees who increase the time they spend on voluntary service activities. However, two change agents are not enough to make much headway in changing organizational values. These two individuals must go down a list of both workplace colleagues and potentially influential outsiders to determine if they should be approached and asked to join a collaborative team.

Other potential recruits should be strongly considered based on the talents they can bring to a collaborative team (Furnham, 2002; et al., 1996). Some individuals are good organizers and can work with people who don't normally care for one another. These individuals are attentive when listening to others, do not become upset with disagreements about peripheral issues, and are skillful in identifying actions that many people may be willing to take. Further, they know enough about the interests of potential collaborators so that they can communicate how their proposal will assist others with *their* causes (Brislin, 2001; Smith, 1988). A mistake change advocates often make is that they search for individuals who agree with them on many issues and who seem sympathetic to the advocates' total collection of causes. This search for like-minded others can cut down too much on the number of people who might collaborate on a specific project. People don't have to agree on everything. They need to agree on the benefits of the one change that the advocates are proposing (Brislin, 2001).

There is another talent that will benefit the developers of organizational change proposals. Some individuals know lots of influential people, that is, they have excellent networks (Gladwell, 2000). If these individuals can be recruited, they can draw on their various contacts in their companies, communities, and professional organizations. Even if they are mid-level managers, these individuals often have good relations with senior executives. They also know journalists, politicians, academics, celebrities, and fund-raisers, all of whom may have contributions to make.

Activists should always keep in mind that there are more and less effective ways to approach senior executives in an organization (Furnham, 2002). Any permanent change will require support "from the top." Change agents should be able to answer questions about "What's in it for me and the organization?" when they meet with the people who will be in charge of the final decision concerning the proposal.

Three other aspects helpful in organizations change will now be discussed. These are goal setting, working with consultants, and recognizing how different sorts of personalities become involved over time when major change efforts are introduced.

Goal Setting. Executives in today's organizations are facing increased competition, often from companies in other countries where labor is cheaper (Kinicki & Williams, 2008). Given this pressure, American executives often find that they must expect more productivity from their workers. Productivity can take many forms. For manufacturing organizations, it can take the form of more units per day, whether the units are shirts, kitchen appliances, computers, or automobiles. For service organizations, productivity takes the form of customers served, potential clients contacted, and ratings of service quality by recent customers.

In attempts to increase productivity, managers and workers can collaborate and set goals for their workplaces (Doest et al., 2006). They can examine past records of production, study what the competition is doing, and then set goals whose achievement will allow the company to stay in business. What form should the goals take? Should managers encourage general goals such as "do your best" or "we need to work harder this year"? Or are specific goals, such as specific numbers of appliances to be produced or potential customers to be contacted, more effective?

Edwin Locke (Locke & Latham, 1984) has carried out extensive research on goal setting and has concluded that goals that involve specific targets are more effective than general goals. He recommends that managers and employees jointly set specific goals and if possible put them in numerical terms. "We will increase revenues by 15 percent" is more effective than "we will sell more products." Some companies use rating scales, and customers rate the service they have received. If a seven-point scale is used, a score of one would indicate very poor service, and a score of seven would indicate excellent service. The goal of "we will increase customer evaluations a full scale point on our seven-point scale" is more effective than "we will serve customers better."

The goals should be challenging. Goals that are too easy to reach will not motivate workers, and goals that are impossible will lead to frustration. The best goals are those that employers and workers feel are challenging and attainable if people focus their efforts and work together so that the specific targets of measurable achievement are reached. As part of the goal setting, specific dates for accomplishment should also be set, such as one month from the present time or a year into the future. People should be given feedback concerning their progress toward goal accomplishment, and they should be rewarded for their successes.

To be effective, goal setting must involve the participation of both employers and workers (Pencavel, 2003; Strauss, 2006). All people in an organization must understand the amount and type of work that will be needed. Further, they must accept the goals as their own and not as burdens imposed on them by unseen company executives. Often, employers will have tentative goals in mind that they bring to a first planning meeting with workers. Some of these employers have been pleasantly surprised when the workers considered these targets and then set even more challenging goals.

As with all forms of workplace participation, there must be a history of trust (Fukuyama, 1995) among employers and workers. In some companies, workers may feel that management has broken promises or has treated previous suggestions for improvement in a cavalier manner. If this is the case, then a new round of participative goal setting is unlikely to increase company performance. With a history of poor employer-worker relations, managers will have to invest time and energy into developing workplace trust. Once trust is established, cooperative goal setting can then be introduced.

Working with Consultants. One reason executives call in outside consultants is that they feel their internal resources are inadequate to deal with pressing problems. Another reason is that executives want specific changes but do not want to be seen as the prime movers behind unpopular decisions. Such decisions may involve reassignments, downsizing, or changes in company direction that affect people's familiar routines. In these cases, consultants are brought in and discover the same problems that management already knows about. The consultants make their recommendations, and the executives can say, "We paid a great deal of money to obtain the views of prestigious outsiders. To be fair to them, we must give their recommendations a chance to be implemented to see if they lead to company improvements."

There are cases of successful consultations that have had a positive impact on organizational success (Carnall, 1990). This discussion will focus on potential difficulties that need to be addressed if consultants are to do good work and if executives and employees will benefit from the resulting recommendations.

Often, consultants are not needed. Many times, employees recognize difficulties and have well-thought approaches to dealing with problems (Strauss, 2006). But executives don't ask their employees and instead bring in consultants. The employees answer the questions posed by consultants and make the same suggestions that they would have told management. The consultants summarize these suggestions, write a report, give it to management, and collect their fees. This leads to the joke told among an organization's employees. "Question: What's the definition of a consultant? Answer: Someone who borrows your watch, tells you what time it is, and charges you for it."

Executives sometimes bring in consultants simply for the dramatic impact that unfamiliar but high-status people may bring (Kahneman & Tversky, 2000). Somehow, it is impressive to fly people from the opposite side of a country, West to East, to give advice. The belief that these fly-in consultants will solve problems is similar to the expectation from folklore that knights in shining armor will come into a village, help the downtrodden and vanquish the oppressors, and then ride off so that people can live happily ever after. Good consultants from the East coast, incidentally, often have to travel to the West coast to have their opinions taken seriously because they then become the glamorous figures arriving at the airport. This leads to two observations. The first is that executives seem to believe that an expert is someone from 3,000 miles away. The second is that consultants often pass each other in mid-air as they fly to each other's cities.

My recommendation is that executives go to the expense of flying in consultants only after working with local expertise. This can start with a questionnaire that is circulated among employees. Assurances of anonymity and the absence of names on a questionnaire can convince employees that their responses are confidential. This recommendation is based on the assumption that, over the years, management and employees have developed trusting relationships (Fukuyama, 1995).

The absence of trust is one reason why the fees of outside consultants must be paid.

Even if executives keep in mind the caveats discussed here, there will be times that they will call in consultants. Without direction from the executives, however, consultants are likely to stumble about and to develop unhelpful recommendations. If they are given the general and unhelpful goal of "suggesting ways for improving the company (Locke & Latham, 1984)," consultants may make recommendations only because they are familiar with certain aspects of organizations. If consultants are well read in organizational structure, they will suggest that the company should reorganize. They will draw impressive-looking organizational charts with arrows indicating who should report to whom. They will also complain that the current structure is unwieldy and that company employees spend too much time writing memos and e-mail messages to each other.

If the consultants have a background in organizational behavior, they will suggest a training program (Aguinis & Kraiger, 2009) aimed at changes in employee behavior. Such training can include better communication skills, sensitivity to people from other cultural groups (Brislin & Yoshida, 1994), or programs dealing with motivation for better customer service. The danger is that the recommended training programs will be "off the shelf." That is, the training will consist of commercially available programs with which the consultants are familiar because they have used them before in other organizations. Such programs may not meet the needs of a specific organization with its unique challenges. One executive recently complained, "Consultants too often have a band-aid that they want to offer my company. Talking with colleagues in other organizations, I find that the same band-aid is being touted as a cure-all for all kinds of problems."

Overly general recommendations that may or may not meet company needs lead to predictable responses from executives. If they find a rose within the thorns, executives can tell employees that they found a recommendation helpful and that they will be making organizational changes. If they do not approve of the recommendations, they can say that the consultants may have good ideas but are unfamiliar with local conditions. Executives will continue, "Given this unfamiliarity, recommendations which might be reasonable in other places are inapplicable here given our unique culture and circumstances."

These potential difficulties, although always a threat, can be lessened if executives are clear about their goals. Rather than ask consultants for the general goal of ways to improve, executives should identify specific targets (Baron and Greenberg, 2008; Locke & Latham, 1984). The best consultations I have seen deal with such specificity: employee classification systems to ensure equitable wages, the integration of Deaf employees into the workplace (Mindess, 1999), and ways of working with the media to improve communications with the general public. Such goal setting allows executives to check on the credentials of potential consultants since specialists often belong to professional organizations where their reputations are well known. Another advantage is that consultants can match up their specific talents with company requirements. Occasionally, consultants will report to company executives that they are not the best people for a certain task and instead will recommend others who have more experience in specific problem areas.

Involving Different Kinds of People in Change Efforts. Organizational innovations require attention to the timing of events and to the different personalities of people who should become involved in change efforts. People often find that they own certain products or hold views on various topics that were unfamiliar or even unthinkable a few years ago. During the 1980s, cell phones were rare and the few who owned them tolerated a technology that is primitive by today's standards. Today, so many people own cell phones that those who don't are sometimes made to feel like relics from the past. When I was a teenager, divorce was a rare event and people talked about it in hushed tones. Today, counseling about the possibility of divorce is part of people's preparation for marriage. Just a few years ago, the music played on American inner-city streets was considered primitive and unsophisticated. Today, rap music is the basis of a multimillion-dollar industry that markets to all parts of the world.

In his book *The Tipping Point*, Malcolm Gladwell (2000) analyzed reasons for the move of products and ideas from the status of unknown to the status of widespread acceptance. He used the term *tipping point* to refer to a combination of people, time, and place that acts like a fulcrum. Imagine a six-foot-long board balancing on a rock with a sharp point that projects upward. If weight is put on the left side of the board, then it will fall in that direction. If weight is put on the other side, that will be the direction of the board's fall. With products and ideas, one side of the board represents ignorance or indifference. The other side represents public awareness and popularity. What tips the balance from one side to the other?

Gladwell (2000) used the language of epidemics in the transmission of disease to analyze the popularization of ideas. One key is that of critical mass. For a flu epidemic to occur, there must be initial carriers who come into contact with other people. Often, these initial carriers have lifestyles that bring them into contact with many other people. For example, street vendors in a crowded market might spread the virus. If these newly infected people come into contact with still others who have no resistance to the disease, then the virus may become well established in a population. Given this critical mass, a flu virus can thrive since it can be continually passed from infected people to previously unaffected ones. If there are no new people who might be infected, the flu virus will cease to be a problem in a population and people will forget about it until they hear about the possibility of a new variant.

With products and concepts such as cell phones, divorce, and rap music, the process is similar in the move from starting point to widespread awareness and acceptance. There is often a small collection of initial figures (Rogers, 2003), such as popular people who start using portable phones. If these people are pictured using their cell phones in magazines such as *People* or *Entertainment Weekly*, this contributes to the reputation that the item is hot. Once these early users spread the message, a second group of people buy and use cell phones. These people are not necessarily well known in a community, but they seem to enjoy and to benefit from the use of their purchases. They spread their experiences by word-of-mouth to members of their social networks. Once a third wave of people begins to buy the product, a critical mass has been reached. Lots of people have cell phones, and their use generates criticism when beepers go off during movies, church services, and the slow and delicate passages of classical music concerts.

Once the third wave of people buys a product, the world seems to be a different place. For example, in the days before everyday access to personal computers, people had to walk to a central processing site to have large amounts of data analyzed. Today, they perform the same analyses on laptop computers. Some readers, along with me, will remember the days when there was a choice among three or four television stations with black-and-white programming. With today's cable television, people can choose among color programming on hundreds of channels.

In the change from products being unfamiliar to becoming widely known and adopted, various types of people play important roles. Gladwell (2000) analyzed how the characteristics of different people combine to make innovation possible. Some people are *visionaries*. They look around their environment and identify unfulfilled needs or possible improvements in existing products (Baron & Tang, 2009). Often, others who do not share the visions label the visionaries as crazy. Visionaries are constantly told, "It can't be done, and you will waste your time and money." Characteristics possessed by successful visionaries include the ability to move beyond conventional thinking and to sort out helpful from discouraging feedback (Baron & Tang, 2009).

After the initial idea is formulated, a group of people known as *connectors* enters the picture. Connectors bring people together. They know lots of people and have good networks in various segments of society

(Brislin, 2001). They are very friendly, and others enjoy hearing that the connectors are trying to reach them and to tell them about their current projects. Since connectors know so many people, they become major figures in word-of-mouth communications about the innovation.

Many innovations involve unfamiliar technologies, and so another group of people enters the picture after connectors stimulate the interest of possible adopters. These technologically sophisticated people are called *mavens* (Gladwell, 2000), and they enjoy telling others about the innovations. Mavens are certainly necessary for the two types of technology being used as examples here. With laptop computers, mavens are needed to help others retrieve programs, link up to the World Wide Web, and to help when data appear to be lost forever. With cable television, mavens are needed to help people use advanced features such as finding out what is showing on hundreds of channels and how to record one program while watching another.

Given the presence of visionaries, connectors, and mavens, new products or ideas begin to become familiar to a small group of enthusiasts. Magazine articles may begin to appear in specialized publications and informal interest groups may form. But the general public is still unconvinced. At this point, salespeople need to enter the picture.

Salespeople have communication skills that allow them to persuade large numbers of people who remain unconvinced. They enjoy talking to others and letting them know about the benefits of the new product. Although not as technologically knowledgeable as mavens, salespeople know basic points about the product and can answer questions about its uses.

Given the activities of these key people, the product then has a chance of disseminating throughout the marketplace. Salespeople are likely to reach a group of people called the *early majority* who are initially skeptical and prefer to observe the reactions of initial product users (Rogers, 2003). If the initial product users engage in enough word-of-mouth enthusiasm, then the majority may give the product a try. Widespread acceptance of a product is marked by frequent comments such as, "How did we ever live without this new product?" People today talk this way about products such as photocopy machines, personal computers, cell phones, and DVD players.

FORMAL TRAINING PROGRAMS

If executives have the goal of constant improvements for the organizations, they make training for employees a central part of their planning (Aguinis & Kraiger, 2009). When deciding that training programs will be offered, executives do not wait for individuals to step forward and to accept or to introduce change efforts. Rather, executives decide that companywide programs are needed that will involve a large number of employees. Training programs must be staffed, organized, and budgeted, and there must be accommodations made for a company's everyday work to be done while different employees are excused from their job responsibilities to attend training programs (Blanchard & Thacker, 2007). The goals of training programs follow an organizational needs assessment including questions such as: What are we doing well? In what areas should we improve? In what areas is our competition outperforming us? Given the increasing demands of our customers and clients, are we serving their needs?

Areas that require improvement are identified from answers to these and similar questions. If improvement is needed in employee and executive attitudes, skills, and behaviors, then a training program could be one part of the change plan (Aguinis & Kraiger, 2009; Blanchard & Thacker, 2007). Training programs are special events that go beyond the day-to-day activities of an organization. They are carefully planned, staffed, and budgeted. Program participants take leave of their regular duties so that they can attend the training program. All these steps mean that there is a considerable investment on the part of management. The trainers must be paid, and the regular duties of the program participants must be assigned to others so that the organization continues to function smoothly.

There are fewer training programs in the United States than there should be. There are more training programs in Asian countries such as Japan, Korea, and Singapore. A major reason is the typical number of years that employees stay with companies in these countries (Triandis, 1995). Although the expectation of lifetime employment with the same company has diminished in Asia, employees engage in less job-hopping than in the United States. Americans change jobs for a wide variety of reasons: better pay, more challenges, desire for a more attractive community, better opportunities for their spouses, more skilled colleagues from whom they can learn, and so forth. Americans read about and have sometimes experienced company downsizing. They believe that their first loyalty is to themselves and to their career development, not to a company whose executives may give them a pink slip at any time.

Employers complain that if they invest in training, there is no guarantee that people will stay with the company. There is no assurance that employees will remain to use the benefits of their training five and six years into the future. Further, the executives complain that employees will rub salt into the wound. They will list the training they received at company A and the skills they developed when they update their resumes as part of their application for a position in company B.

Training can involve a significant investment of organizational resources (Blanchard & Thacker, 2007). It is indeed frustrating to see one's well-trained employees now working for a competitor. But as one wise executive said, "Yes, it is expensive to train employees who later leave the company. But given that potential customers have many choices of where to do business, it is more expensive to have untrained employees who stay with the company."

Decisions about Training Programs. When an organization's executives engage in strategic planning, they set goals and then decide how to achieve them (Locke & Latham, 1984). If one path toward achieving the goals is to increase employee skills, then executives have a number of options. They can send employees to classes at a nearby university. They can encourage on-the-job training where knowledgeable employees pass on their skills to others. If the organization has a human resources department, its staff members can be asked to prepare an on-site training program. Or, the executives can contract with a company that specializes in training, and the program can be held off-site at a conference center.

Whatever the choice, executives should specify the desired program content. Assume professional trainers, either in-house or contracted from the outside, are asked to design a program. If given only general guidelines, trainers will often adapt a program that they have previously used or have seen done at another organization. The danger with such "off-the-shelf" programs is that they do not always meet the specific needs and specific goals of the organization that is paying for the training (Ellis, Bell, Ployhart, Hollenbeck, & Ilgen, 2005). Good trainers can take a list of topics that executives want covered and then design a new program that becomes an important part of the organization's strategic planning.

Good programs contain material on awareness of company goals, necessary new knowledge, emotional challenges, and actual behaviors that employees incorporate into their everyday interactions (Brislin & Yoshida, 1994). As an example, assume the organization has decided to market its products to Deaf consumers and to hire more Deaf employees. Trainees will be employees who interact daily with customers. Awareness training introduces the employees to Deaf culture (Mindess, 1999). A major part of the culture is American Sign Language, which is not simply a collection of gestures. It is a fully developed, complex language that requires years of study and practice if people are to become fluent. Knowledge includes ways of communicating more effectively. Note-passing among Deaf and hearing people is common, and hearing people can develop an elementary knowledge of sign language. If nothing else, being able to use a few signs will make the Deaf feel more welcome. Another piece of knowledge is that the Deaf have asked people to capitalize the word when referring to their culture, just as we capitalize American and Greek when referring to those cultures.

Trainers cover emotional challenges that could interfere with strategic goals if not well understood. The Deaf do not like the term *hearing impaired* since people may interpret it as brain damage or as an imposed limitation on their interactions in society. The Deaf sometimes ask, "Why can't we call you signing impaired?" Actual behaviors need to be incorporated into people's everyday repertoires. For communications that need to go beyond basic signing and notes, an interpreter will be required. A hearing person should keep eye contact with and be attentive to the Deaf person, even though there is a temptation to direct one's communication at the interpreter who is speaking (Mindess, 1999). If people practice new behaviors, they will eventually become habitual and will increase communication effectiveness.

Decisions about Timing in Training Programs. There is no question that training demands an investment of company resources. Given the costs, there is a temptation to cram as much information in a training program as possible, but this tactic may work against company goals (Chiaburu & Marinova, 2005). This is an issue in this incident.

The Timing of Workplace Training Is Important

"We will be investing a lot of money in this training program, but I think it will pay for itself in the long run through increased business," Bill Jeffords told his staff. Bill was the president of a company that sold office supplies. To differentiate his company from his competitors, Bill wanted to introduce a delivery system direct from his warehouse to the desks of people who purchased from him. This innovation meant that all members of his staff would have to be trained in an information management system that would track orders from customers. The system would allow Bill to tell customers the status of orders, when they would be delivered, and when it was necessary to restock the warehouse.

Bill signed a contract with an organization that offered training programs in information technology management. He felt it would be most efficient if a large percentage of his workers took the 16-hour program over two days. He would keep a skeleton crew of recent college graduates, who had previously taken courses in information technology and so had less need for the training, to handle orders during the two days.

The training program seemed to go well. Workers were enthusiastic and seemed to be learning a great deal. When Bill stopped by to see how the program was going, he was pleased to see that his workers had animated facial expressions and were studying hard. At the end of the program, workers rated the program highly, saying that the trainers were well prepared and were able to answer specific questions. The trainers reported back to Bill that they thought that participants learned the material and that the goals of the program were accomplished.

However, a month later, the company was making little progress in its efforts to introduce the new technology. Workers made a lot of mistakes that caused orders to go to the wrong customer. People frequently complained that they had forgotten important material covered during the program. In fact, the workers who were able to use the technology most efficiently were the recent college graduates who did not attend the training program.

Bill's company is the victim of a problem with training programs that are squeezed into a full day or more. People's memories are fallible, and they simply forget a great deal of material that is crammed into an eight-hour day (Chiaburu & Marinova, 2005). They also can become fatigued, and this affects their memories. Training is much more effective, with long-term retention of material, when it is spaced over more days (Baddeley, Eysenck, & Anderson, 2009). If Bill could have scheduled the program so that workers could attend two hours for each of eight days, participants would not forget as much material. One reason why the college graduates were able to use the technology is that they learned their skills over a longer period of time. Typically, college students spend three hours a week in class for 15 weeks. With this schedule, they have time to think about their new learning and to ask questions about material covered in earlier sessions. Such a schedule also allows them to do homework assignments that reinforce their classroom learning.

Training programs that cram material into long sessions are more popular than programs spread over many days. One reason is that scheduling is easier. If employees leave their offices to attend a training program, their regular work needs to be covered by others. It is easier to do this for long programs that consume a few days than it is for programs spread over many days. In addition, there is a great deal of enthusiasm during full day programs. Participants think they are learning a great deal and report this at the end-of-session evaluations (K. Brown, 2005). Only later does the fallibility of memory take its toll as workers find they have forgotten a great deal of material from the program (Baddeley et al., 2009).

INDIVIDUAL DIFFERENCES IN THE ACCEPTANCE OF CHANGE

Different people have various reasons for accepting, rejecting, or actively sabotaging change efforts in their organizations. In addition, some people may seem to accept change, but will behave according to the change only under limited circumstances (Kelman, 1958; 2006). The difference between real and ersatz acceptance of change is an issue in this incident.

Motives Differ for Those Who Accept Change

"We run low on key items that our customers need," Alan Percy told his employees. "We need a more efficient tracking system for the products we sell so that we can replace them from our warehouses." Alan was the manager of a building supplies company that sold directly to contractors. He felt that he was disappointing too many customers who left his store without the products they needed, and that he was losing too much business to his competitors. He felt that change was needed. So he introduced a new tracking system for items sold that was based on the use of small hand-held computers. He organized training sessions during which employees learned to use the computers.

Three months after the new system was introduced, Alan called a meeting with his employees so that he could receive feedback about the changes. Afterward, Alan commented to his assistant, "People seem to be using the computers, but I get the feeling that not all of them are doing it for the same reason."

Alan is probably correct. People follow the directives of authority figures for various reasons. Herbert Kelman (1958; 2006) has investigated three reasons:

1. Compliance: People accept the directives of authority figures so they will gain rewards and avoid punishments. But they don't necessarily think that the directives are reasonable or helpful.
2. Identification: People change their behavior—in this case use of the small computers—because they desire a positive relationship with the authority figure who issues the directives.
3. Internalization: People change their behavior because they genuinely feel it is wise to do so and that they will be better employees if they follow the lead of their managers.

Compliance may be the easiest to understand since everyone engages in some behaviors to gain rewards and to avoid punishments (Baddeley et al., 2009). Children learn not to play in the street to gain the approval of their parents and to avoid disapproval. Employees accept some company directives to reap rewards such as salary increases, promotions, and the approval of managers. But if employees are following directives only because of compliance, they will behave in ways of their own choosing if they no longer receive any rewards.

A new manager may introduce another tracking system, and employees are likely to use it, if accepting the new directives leads to rewards.

When people change their behavior because of identification, they do so because they respect the person who suggests the change. They might say to themselves, "We wouldn't adopt the new tracking system if it was up to us, but Alan has been a good manager. We want to have good relationships with him. Let's give his suggestions a try out of respect for him." The danger with change due to identification is that it is tied to one individual. If Alan leaves the organization, employees may abandon his policies.

With internalization, people change because they think that the directives of authority figures are consistent with their personal values, such as the importance of customer service (McGuire, 1985). They will continue to use the innovative method because they are convinced that company goals are being met more efficiently. In the case of the tracking system, employees will use the system even if Alan leaves. Further, if the employees move to another organization, they might suggest using the same technology to their new managers. With internalization, people behave in ways that they think about in positive terms such as valuable, efficient, helpful, and intelligent (Park et al., 2007; Petty et al., 2003).

All three change processes can occur after authority figures issue a directive. Especially during their first months on a job, employees might use a new tracking system just to avoid the punishment of being terminated during their probationary periods. They might show more enthusiasm about using the system if they discover that their manager usually makes good decisions. Then, they might internalize use of the system if they discover that it makes them good employees who are better able to serve their customers. Another aspect of change programs is the intelligence level of the people toward whom efforts are being addressed (Petty et al., 2003). Many times, people underestimate the intelligence of the people in their organizations. They only cover the arguments in favor of change and do not give their audience enough credit to consider the advantages and disadvantages of the recommended change.

People stand up in front of others and voice their opinions about change for a variety of reasons. They may want to show their support for a new company policy. They may want to endorse or derogate a candidate campaigning for a union position or argue the merits of a proposed workplace regulation. They may want to condemn recent executive decisions that they think are unfair. They may want to urge others to act in certain ways, such as to form a union in their organization. Often, when people decide to speak in public, they want others to change certain attitudes. But the others may have very well established attitudes and thus efforts to encourage change will be difficult (Sherif et al., 1965).

I sometimes watch public access television shows that cover community forums such as the city council, hearings at the state capitol, or various neighborhood boards. People stand up and speak in the hopes of persuading others about community issues, but they often behave as if they have no knowledge of persuasive communication (Cortes, 2000; Martin, 1999; McGuire, 1985). The speakers present their message and are clear about their own position. Then, people on the other side of the issue stand and give their position. Many times, voices become loud and the choice of vocabulary becomes highly emotional. In such cases, there is no two-way communication. People are simply talking to like-minded people and are not making attempts to reach out to others who disagree. The others may behave in the same way, preaching their position to supporters who happen to be at the meeting, and again there is no real communication. These meetings often end with people convinced that their position is correct, just as they were at the beginning of the meeting.

Good persuasive communication that may contribute to attitude change involves knowing the position of others who disagree and reaching out to them (Petty & Brinol, 2008). It involves knowledge of others, the challenges of changing their attitudes, and respect for their ideas. There are various steps that people can take if they hope to change attitudes. One step is to engage in two-sided communication (Jones & Brehm, 1970). Instead of presenting just one side of the issue, good speakers point out the positive aspects of opponents' positions. This is especially true when others who disagree are intelligent and well informed. If people take the trouble to leave their homes and to attend community meetings, it is a good assumption that they possess these assets.

Two-sided communications have many advantages. Let's use the example of universal health care. Side A is that there should be a national health insurance plan administered by the government. Side B is that health insurance should be left to the private sector. People advocating for side A in the United States have to be persuasive to change attitudes because there is no national health care insurance program for all people. If they engage in two-sided communication, speakers advocating side A must be knowledgeable about various positions surrounding the issue. This means that they will be much better prepared when they present their recommendations.

Advocates of side A should recognize points emphasized by side B, such as the risk of a massive government bureaucracy. People in favor of side B will respect the speakers for taking the trouble to recognize the positive aspects of their position (Aronson, Wilson, & Akert, 2010;

McGuire, 1985). They may reciprocate by acknowledging the positive points presented by the proponents, such as better health care for the economically disadvantaged. Now we have communication! People are beginning to move away from speaking only to the like-minded and are reaching out to others. When the advantages and disadvantages of various positions are recognized, there is a greater chance of developing a compromise position that will be acceptable to both sides. If this takes place, everyone adjusts their attitudes a little bit so that a workable policy can be formulated.

14

Some Final Considerations

Given that people spend so much of their lives in the world of work, it is not surprising to find the wide range of issues that they will encounter in their quest for workplace satisfaction. People meet others who are more and less capable, who are more and less thoughtful, who have a variety of personalities, who have very different social skills, and who come from diverse backgrounds. People must develop a variety of skills and must possess a great deal of knowledge to navigate the myriad issues they will encounter. In this final chapter, I would like to discuss some key points from various previous chapters that I feel are especially important for finding workplace satisfaction. These points are based on my reading of the scholarly literature, on discussions with colleagues, from attendance at professional meetings, from interviews with workers in a variety of fields, and from my own work experience in a variety of settings inside and outside of academia.

LEADERSHIP

People enjoy working for leaders who have a clear vision; managers with leadership ambitions have more success when they are able to describe a better future that incorporates their ideas and contributions. A vision involves a clear outcome, not unlike a painting that clearly depicts a lush landscape or an exciting street scene. In addition to the vision, leaders need to indicate the steps that others need to take so that the vision is realized. The steps need to be clearly communicated so that listeners, who are most often a company's employees, will see how they fit into plans for the future and what actions they must take to contribute to the goals specified in the vision.

People appreciate leaders who are concerned with the welfare of employees. This can take different forms depending on the personalities of leaders. Some leaders show concern by leading a company with such expertise and competence that workers realize their company is likely to prosper. Other leaders will show concern though consideration of employee feelings and will take steps to ensure that good workers are appreciated and rewarded. Some leaders can combine both approaches. Some leaders realize that they have one of the skills sets, task competence or employee consideration, but not the other. If this is the case, they are well advised to select assistants who can complement their abilities.

Leaders must be sensitive to the social contexts in which they find themselves. Different contexts, or collections of situations, are influenced by actions such as the performance of competitors, changes in the demographic characteristics of customers, changing market conditions, employee concerns given their knowledge of current company financial performance, and so forth. To achieve the status of respected leaders, people need to be aware of various topics covered in this book, such as communication, attitude change, power, social skills, and organizational change. Leaders need to know that they will be looked at for cues as to how employees should behave to both contribute to company goals and to achieve approval from leaders.

GROUPS

People reap extensive benefits from their membership in groups, and they enjoy being valued members of groups and are extremely uncomfortable when they are excluded or shunned. From their group memberships, people receive help on complex tasks, learn about opportunities in their organizations and their communities, and receive social support in times of stress. There is little doubt that people have a need for human contact and for pleasant interactions with others. Few of us would enjoy being hermits.

The need for human contact and group membership stems from prerecorded history. People who were valued members of groups received food when they were hungry, water when they were thirsty, and shelter when they experienced bad weather. Loners who tried to solve such needs on their own were less likely to survive. The strong peer group influences every parent observes in their adolescent children is a result of benefits that fell to group members long ago. In prerecorded history, many adolescents were orphans.

Groups can bring benefits to people, but they can also bring troubles. People can be pressured to conform to the incorrect opinions of a majority, even if they are convinced that the majority is wrong. Rather than stand out from the group and maintain an individual independent voice, many people will go along with the group so that they are not seen as deviants. People can also be swayed by the opinions of group members, a process known as *groupthink*. Problems can occur when a group is tightly knit and members enjoy each other's company, but they are faced with challenging issues about which they must make decisions. In discussions about the issues, there is pleasure when other people seem to agree with commonly held opinions. Given this apparent agreement, there is no search for alternative opinions that might cause people to reconsider or to sharpen their original position. An individual who speaks up with a dissenting opinion is often ridiculed.

Group efforts can also bring benefits. Group members can set challenging goals that will improve their organization, and they can assist each other in goal accomplishment. More work can be accomplished by five people working cooperatively than those same five people working by themselves. The challenge for leaders is to recognize the power of groups and to guide them into productivity rather than destructive groupthink efforts.

COGNITIONS

People think a great deal about events in their lives. They ponder their futures and decide whether or not investments in more education will pay various types of dividends. They plan for the futures of their children. People consider whether or not to stay with their current organization or to seek employment elsewhere. After considering various potential difficulties in their lives, they conclude that they can handle some well but will be stressed by others. People will twist and turn their internal cognitions so that they appear to be reasonable people both to themselves and to others.

Some collections of thoughts are based on comparisons with others. People do not always compare themselves with absolute standards, such as salaries given certain titles in an organization or the size and splendor of their homes. Rather, they compare themselves with others who are much like themselves with regard to the lifestyle they want to experience. People in a small Midwestern community do not compare themselves to people in Boston. They compare themselves with others in similar-sized communities. They often stretch their thinking to put themselves in a favorable light. They may not drive a Porsche or a

BMW like several of their neighbors, but they are proud of the amount of time they spend with their children.

Whether or not people become stressed is influenced by their cognitions. People think about potential difficulties and decide whether they are bothered by them or not. For some people, public speaking is a stressor and for some it is not. After the cognitions surrounding this first analysis, people decide whether they can cope with the potential stress. If they know how to use PowerPoint, or if they have friends who can help with the public presentation, their stress may be reduced significantly. Finally, they can decide whether the stress is worth the threat to their health and well-being. This step is often facilitated by colleagues and counselors. These helpers ask, "Is it really worth your energy to get upset about an upcoming speech you are expected to give? There are so many other more important problems that need your attention and your talents!"

COMMUNICATION DIFFICULTIES

So people think a great deal about their behavior. What happens when they enter the workplace? They must think about themselves as well as others with whom they come into contact. When multiple people interact, trying to share their cognitions about current events, they are likely to have communication difficulties with others who are also wedded to their cognitions.

There are various biases that have been identified when people communicate, and people must give attention to these potential stumbling blocks if they are to achieve ambitious workplace goals. One communication difficulty is called the *confirmation bias*. People have their opinions, and then they examine information in their environment and cherry-pick those perceived facts that will support their opinion. People are not skillful at considering their opinions as tentative hypotheses that should be examined by looking at both supportive and unsupportive information. People then share their opinions that are reinforced by the confirmation bias. They may be on a selection committee and have negative views about a certain candidate based on experiences from 10 years ago. When they read a letter of recommendation, they are likely to jump at phrases they perceive as negative and to downplay positive paragraphs. When they share their opinions, they may be surprised to find that others did not interpret the selected phrases in such a negative manner.

The *self-serving bias* is based on the fact that most people think of themselves as decent individuals who have a lot to offer to their organizations. If they don't feel this way and feel that they are not worthwhile individuals, then they are showing a sign of a depressed mental state. This self-serving bias contributes to people's feelings that they work harder than their parents and their grandparents. Everyone else they meet says that they are so busy that they have no time for themselves! If people are to maintain a positive self-image, they may not want to think of themselves as lazy loafers who value their leisure time. Rather, they are likely to join in the conversation and to complain about all the demands on their time.

Effective Communication. After studying the research on communication biases, people might conclude that efforts to speak with others will lead to disasters. People should certainly be aware of communication biases, and they can also be assisted if they are aware of various contributions that have been offered by behavioral researchers. These contributions are especially helpful to have in mind when people attempt to communicate with others who are different in terms of age, culture, gender, and social class.

The distinction between high- and low-context communication is important. Discussion of this distinction brings up a theme that has been covered several times in this book: People must be aware of the situational influences on their behavior and that of others. In high-context communication, the information is contained in the message and associated cues that people are supposed to understand. The phrase "supposed to understand" means that people share a background where the cues attached to a message are learned. A husband and wife, married for 30 years, can glance at each other three hours into a party and can conclude that both are bored and that it is time to say their goodbyes. Their communication is high-context. It does not have to be carefully and elaborately verbalized. In contrast, two people who have been dating for two months would have difficulty communicating with a mere glance. They would have to meet in a corner, discuss explicitly their feelings about the party, and then make a decision concerning whether to leave or not. This is low-context communication: The intent of a message must be carefully spelled out.

The fact that both the married and dating couples are exchanging glances is a reminder of the importance of nonverbal communication. Often, the meaning that a recipient takes away from a communication event is largely based on nonverbal cues that accompany the sender's choice of vocabulary. Nonverbal cues include body posture, voice tone, amount of eye contact, number and magnitude of hand gestures, and so forth. These nonverbal cues are often shared among people who have the same background in terms of culture, age, and social class. If people are communicating with others who have different backgrounds, they should make efforts to ensure that the nonverbal part of their message is understood. An unthinking belief that "If I want to communicate a message, it will be received by others" should be replaced by a more careful analysis of the total context surrounding one's communication attempts.

UNDERSTANDING POWER

People with power have more access to an organization's resources than others who are powerless. Resources include good-paying jobs, prestigious automobiles, high-status home addresses, access to influential community members, the admiration of others, and company perks such as business-class travel. Given the importance of resources for survival and for a comfortable life, some people take power seriously and learn strategies and tactics for its use. People can consider joining the ranks of sophisticated power seekers, or they can seek out power-oriented individuals for collaborative interactions. Powerful people are useful to have on one's side. They can be good friends but can also be bad enemies.

Strategies for the use of power include dividing one's work into winnable steps. Then, when a step is achieved, people come across as winners who can get things done. They don't communicate the message that they are "losers" who can be counted on to stumble and fail. When people have the image of winners, others want to join their efforts so that they can bask in the glow of success. This fact is summarized in a commonly heard phrase: Everyone loves a winner.

Other strategies center on the acquisition of resources. Since power involves resources, people who have a resource can trade it for others in the quest for status and influence. Resources include money, information, goods, and services. Young adults with a hefty trust fund have an advantage. They can invest money in various community causes, meeting powerful people in the process. If the young adults make it clear that they have money to donate and to invest, others will beat paths toward their doors. For people without money, information from their formal and informal education is most often their resource. If they have information powerful people need, such as tax accounting, medical knowledge, or legal expertise, they will find themselves in the company of influential individuals.

SOCIAL SKILLS

A discussion of power might stimulate readers to run to a library and check out the writings of Machiavelli. This could be a good idea, but it is not if readers feel that they have to adopt manipulative tactics summarized by the term *Machiavellianism*. Powerholders are often very socially skilled, charming, and gracious people. Since power involves influence over others, socially skilled people have an advantage because others are more willing to defer to likable than unlikable people. This is especially true in a democracy where people have some choices about designating who is powerful, but it is also true in totalitarian societies where tyrannical leaders can eventually wear out their welcome if they are abusive with their power.

Social skills refer to people's ability to interact smoothly with others such that the others feel good and look forward to future interactions. Socially skilled people can develop networks of powerful and influential individuals. Powerholders appreciate the presence of socially skilled people who can contribute to a pleasant, optimistic, and forward-looking set of norms for formal organizations as well as more informal community volunteer activities. The development of social skills for today's workplace activities can begin with memories of what our parents tried to teach us. They told us to listen respectfully to others, to take turns, to share with others, and to not always be the center of attention.

Other social skills take practice. People should learn to accept criticism graciously. Even if they would like to shout at critics, they will develop a more positive community image if they remain calm and thank the critics for their suggestions. The ability to accept criticism follows from the development of a thick skin. People who rise to the top of their organizations will be the targets of criticism. There will always be others who feel that they should have been chosen for a promotion or that their suggestions for a policy change should have been accepted. Influential people have to realize that receiving criticism is part of their jobs. Many times, younger people concerned with the thinness of their skins can take steps to move toward armadillo-like status. They can join community groups, thus increasing the size of their networks, and join a committee where people will surely disagree. In my experience, people on a group's budget committee are sure to receive criticism no matter what they recommend concerning use of the group's funds.

ATTITUDES

Attitudes refer to people's evaluation reactions to social objects in their lives including cognitions (what they think the important facts are) and behavioral tendencies to approach or to avoid those social objects. Some attitudes are relatively unimportant in people's lives. For example, they may not care much for Mexican or Thai food, but they can tolerate it. Because they do not have strong attitudes, they may defer to the wishes of their lunch companions if they have a strong preference for one ethnic cuisine over the other. Ego-involved attitudes are important to people's sense of self-identity and to the image they want to project to others. People can have strong attitudes that they are willing to express forcefully on issues such as leadership, religion, the proper role of government, economic policy, and the importance of higher education for one's children. These ego-involved attitudes do not change easily.

One way to measure ego-involved attitudes is to consider people's latitudes, or areas, of acceptance, rejection, and neutrality. Latitudes of acceptance include cognitions, feelings, or behavioral tendencies that are consistent with a person's general position on an important issue. If people have strong attitudes about the importance of work in their lives, they will find hard-working others, merit pay, and work incentives in their latitude of acceptance. They will find lazy people and colleagues who only invest the minimum in their jobs to be in the latitude of rejection. There may be aspects of work about which they are neutral: the length of their lunch hour, parking, and paperwork for travel reimbursements can be examples. Often, if others communicate with people who have ego-involved attitudes, verbalizations that come close to the latitude of acceptance may be pulled in and included in people's thinking about the communicator and the communication. In addition, verbalizations that come close to the latitude of rejection may be rejected as unreasonable or poorly thought out, again affecting thinking about the communicator.

Positive attitudes bring great benefits to people. Others enjoy being in their presence and communicating with them. As a result, the people learn a great deal about what is going on in their organizations, communities, and professions. Positive attitudes also contribute to organizational citizenship. Positive people are likely to take on tasks that are not specifically detailed in their job descriptions. As a result, they develop exchange relations with others who will pitch in when the good organizational citizens need help. The efforts of good organizational citizens are also remembered when company executives consider promotions and pay raises.

DECISION MAKING

In organizational decision making, a major issue is whether time, energy, and resources should be spent on the decision-making process or whether a quick decision is "good enough." Executives cannot spend all the time they might want on every decision. They have to make a judgment concerning whether the decision area is central to the organization, demanding time and energy, or whether a less careful decision will lead to satisfactory outcomes.

Often, quick decision making is based on heuristics. There are guidelines to decisions that quickly come to mind. One guideline is the availability heuristic. Some decisions have suggested solutions that come quickly to mind and can be easily retrieved from memory. One result of an availability heuristic might be, "We have always had good performance from interns sent by a nearby university. Let's continue with them this year." Other heuristics are captured by adages, such as "A stitch in time saves nine." Applying this heuristic to a current organizational problem, a leader might say, "Let's give this seemingly small problem some attention now so that it does not lead to major difficulties in the future."

If executives decide that they must engage in careful analysis before making a decision, there are a number of tools available. One is a SWOT (strengths, weaknesses, opportunities, and threats) analysis that executives can consider surrounding potential decisions. For example, executives might be considering expansion of their products and services into new markets. Strengths could include the company's brand image and the high quality of their workforce. Weaknesses could include the need to hire more people in a sinking economic situation that does not allow the hiring of the many new employees who are needed for expansion. Opportunities could include the opening of international markets that were closed in the recent past. Threats will always include the actions of competitors. If expansion into new markets is seen as desirable by one company, it may be seen as desirable by several.

WORKER MOTIVATION

When managers are concerned with worker motivation, they are interested in the movement of people toward the accomplishment of goals valued by the organization. There is a difference between motivation and morale, even though the terms are often used interchangeably. Motivation is a concept applied to individuals. If individuals work hard toward the achievement of company goals, then they are said to be motivated. Morale is a concept applied to groups of people. If people value their organization, appreciate their colleagues, and feel that they are contributing to group goals, they are said to have a high level of morale.

All theories of motivation have a concept known as *valences*. The term refers to what workers want from their organizations. Different workers have different combinations of valences. Typical valences include money, cordial coworkers, appreciation from supervisors, opportunities for skill development and promotions, and the possibility of making contributions to one's profession that become known outside one's organization. Attention to money as a valence has increased over the last 50 years. People need more money to buy the seeming necessities that did not exist 50 years ago: home computers, cell phones, digital televisions with their

500+ channels, a car for each family member over 16 years of age, and so forth. The importance of a college education for career success has increased, leading to tuition bills for parents and grandparents. Workers are quick to change jobs if they feel that they can do better financially in another organization, and executives should take pains to make sure that their salary structures are competitive.

Workers want equity in the satisfaction of their valences. They want to be able to look at their contributions to their workplace and feel that the benefits they receive are consistent with those contributions. They also want to be able to look at other people, with whom they are familiar, and see that they are receiving similar outcomes (pay, benefits) if they are producing as much on their jobs. Feelings of inequity lead to the quest for a new job in another organization.

An especially important fact about motivation and valences is that workers will always want more. They will go through their lists of valences and decide whether or not they are being satisfied in the workplace. If they feel they are receiving adequate salaries, they will turn their attention to their benefits. If they feel that their benefits are competitive with other organizations, they will turn their attention to other valences such as cordial colleagues or opportunities for skill development through advanced training. Workers will never be satisfied. If they receive good outcomes, they will become participants in "a revolution of rising expectations" and will look for other positive outcomes. This is an example of human nature about which managers should familiarize themselves.

OVERCOMING PREJUDICE, EMBRACING DIVERSITY

Many developments in society have contributed to the reduction of prejudice in the United States, and many other countries, over the last 75 years. Organizations cannot afford to alienate members of any group as customers. Laws require adherence to equal opportunities for all people. Standards of common decency dictate that people be allowed to pursue happiness regardless of skin color, religion, sexual orientation, or other factors that previously led to discrimination.

Prejudice is a type of attitude directed against groups other than one's own. Although there are occasionally positive prejudices, such as a romantic feeling toward people in another culture who seem to be leading a purer life, the term is most used in reference to negative feelings. These feelings take various forms. With intense racism, people from one group feel that members of another are inferior by the fact of their birth. Intense racism is very resistant to change. In contrast to intense racism, there is a greater chance of changing prejudices based on likes and dislikes and on unfamiliar behaviors. People in some cultures engage in behaviors that other people dislike. Nepotism in hiring practices is an example. In some cultures, this is a way of contributing to one's collective and taking care of others for whom one has responsibilities. In other cultures, the practice denies opportunities to qualified individuals not blessed by favorable kin relations. Unfamiliar behaviors need to be explained, and such explanations can often lessen the feelings associated with prejudice. The need to be indirect and non-confrontational in a receiver-oriented culture makes sense because people have been socialized to figure out the meaning behind messages without direct and detailed communications.

Executives can take steps to reduce prejudices in their organizations and can insist that energies once invested in discrimination now be put into positive efforts that will contribute to company growth. They can take steps to ensure that all employees have equal status in the organization, with corresponding opportunities for the best jobs, promotions, and benefits. They can introduce superordinate goals that are valued by all employees and that clearly need the efforts of all to ensure goal accomplishment. They can support the encouragement of multiple identities. One aspect of employee self-identity will always be, "I am a member of a certain ethnic or cultural group." But another identity can be, "I am a member of an organization that values cultural diversity and that values my contributions."

CHANGE

People become accustomed to their daily routine and when they do not encounter major difficulties, they see little reason to change. If adjustments to the status quo are necessary, leaders have to communicate why the future will see improvements if changes are adopted. Goal setting is a powerful tool. Leaders, with suggestions from employees, can set goals that are challenging and yet still attainable with high levels of effort. Leaders can communicate company goals, and then ask individual employees to formulate their own plans for the future with the goals in mind. Goals should be specific. If employees agree to increase sales, a specific number of potential new customers should be targeted. The goal should not be the more general, "increase the number of customers who utilize our products and services."

Over time, employees can seem to accept the change recommended by leaders, or they can genuinely accept it. If they comply with change, they will behave according to the recommendations only because they want to obtain the rewards or avoid any punishers that their leaders control. If they change through the process known as *identification*, they will accept recommendations because they like, respect, or appreciate the efforts of the leaders. The difficulty is that if the leaders leave the organization, there will no longer be any reason to behave according to the recommendations. If employees internalize the changes, they do so because the changes clearly lead to improvements. Employees genuinely feel that they are making more contributions to their organizations, and they will continue to behave according to the recommendations even if the leaders leave.

And this leads us back to the major theme of the book. I hope that people can internalize beliefs surrounding the goal, "I can find happiness and satisfaction in my workplace. Specifically, I can get up in the morning and look forward to leaving my home and going to work." I hope they can internalize thoughts such as, "I am knowledgeable about cognitions, attitudes, communication, and groups in the workplace. I know that many individuals are power-oriented, but I am sophisticated enough and know enough about power to deal with these individuals. I know enough about the benefits of diversity and the need for major adjustments given changes in markets, competitors, and customer demographics." If people are able to increase the sophistication of their thinking and behavior on these topics, they will become important contributors to their organizations and will reap the benefits that such status brings.

References

Abelson, R. (1981). Psychological status of the script concept. *American Psychologist*, 36, 715–729.

Adams, J. (1965). Inequity in social exchange. In *Advances in experimental social psychology*, Vol. 2, ed. L. Berkowitz, 267–299. New York: Academic Press.

Adler, N. (2002). *International dimensions of organizational behavior* (4th ed.). Boston: PWS-Kent.

Aguinis, H., & Kraiger, K. (2009). Benefits of training and development for individuals and teams, organizations, and society. *Annual Review of Psychology*, 60, 451–474.

Allen, M., & Preiss, R. (Eds.) (1998). *Persuasion: Advances through meta-analysis*. Cresskill, NJ: Hampton Press.

Allen, T., Finkelstein, L., & Poteet, M. (2009). *Designing workplace mentoring programs: An evidence-based approach*. New York: Wiley-Blackwell.

Allport, G. (1954). *The nature of prejudice*. Reading, MA: Addison-Wesley.

Allport, G., & Postman, L. (1945). The basic psychology of rumor. *Proceedings of the New York Academy of Sciences, Series II, VIII*, 61–81.

Amir, Y. (1969). Contact hypothesis in ethnic relations. *Psychological Bulletin, 71*, 319–343.

Amy, A. (2008). Leaders as facilitators of individual and organizational learning. *Leadership & Organization Development Journal, 29*, 212–234.

Aosved, A., Long, P., & Voller, E. (2009). Measuring sexism, racism, sexual prejudice, ageism, classism, and religious intolerance: The Intolerant Schema Measure. *Journal of Applied Social Psychology, 39*, 2321–2354.

Aparna, J. (2006) The influence of organizational demography on the external networking behavior of teams. *Academy of Management Review, 31*, 583–595.

Aronson, E., & Patnoe, S. (1997). *The jigsaw classroom* (2nd ed.). New York: Longman.

Aronson, E., Wilson, T., & Akert, R. (2010). *Social psychology*, 7th ed. Boston: Prentice Hall.

Asch, S. (1956). Studies of independence and conformity: A minority of one against unanimous majority. *Psychological Monographs, 70* (Whole No. 416).

Ashmore, R., Deaux. K., & McLaughlin-Volpe, T. (2004). An organizing framework for collective identity: Articulation and significance of multidimensionality. *Psychological Bulletin, 130,* 80–114.

Atran, S., & Axelrod, R. (2008). Reframing sacred values. *Negotiation Journal, 24,* 221–246.

Attardo, S. (1997). The semantic foundations of cognitive theories of humor. *Humor—International Journal of Humor Research, 10,* 395–420.

Aycan, Z. (2008). Cross-cultural approaches to leadership. In *The handbook of cross-cultural management research*, eds. P. Smith, M. Peterson, & D. Thomas, 219–238. Thousand Oaks, CA: SAGE.

Baddeley, A., Eysenck, M., & Anderson, M. (2009). *Memory*. New York: Psychology Press.

Bandura, A. (2001). Social cognitive theory: An agentive perspective. *Annual Review of Psychology, 52,* 1–26.

Baretto, M., Ryan, M., & Schmitt, M. (Eds.) (2009). *The glass ceiling in the 21st century: Understanding barriers to gender equality.* Washington, DC: American Psychological Association.

Barna, L. (2009). The stress dynamic and its intersection with intercultural communication. In *Contemporary leadership and intercultural competence: Exploring the cross-cultural dynamics within organizations,* ed. M. Moodian, 139–144. Thousand Oaks, CA: SAGE.

Baron, R., & Tang, J. (2009). Entrepreneurs' social skills and new venture performance: Mediating mechanisms and cultural generality. *Journal of Management, 35,* 282–306.

Baumeister, R. (2005). *The cultural animal: Human nature, meaning, and social life.* New York: Oxford University Press.

Baumeister, R., & Vohs, K. (2007). Self-regulation, ego depletion, and motivation. *Social and Personality Psychology Compass, 1,* 115–128.

Baumeister, R., Vohs, K., & Funder, D. (2007). Psychology as the science of self-reports and finger movements: Whatever happened to actual behavior? *Perspectives on Psychological Science, 2,* 396–403.

Bays, G. (2007). Let's talk: Preparing students for speaking and listening in the workplace. In *Resources in technical communication: Outcomes and approaches,* ed. C. Selfe, 281–291. Amityville, NY: Baywood Publishing.

Bem, D. (1972). Self-perception theory. In *Advances in experimental social psychology*, Vol. 6, ed. L. Berkowiz, 1–62. New York: Academic Press.

Bernstein, B. (1971). *Class, codes and control*, Vol. 1. London: Paladin.

Beyer, J., Chattopadhyay, P., George, E., Glick, W., & Pugliese, D. (1997). The selective perception of managers revisited. *Academy of Management Journal, 40,* 716–737.

Blass, T. (2004). *The man who shocked the world: The life and legacy of Stanley Milgram.* New York: Basic Books.

Bianci, S., Robinson, J., & Milkie, M. (2006). *Changing rhythms of American family life*. New York: Russell Sage Foundation.

Blanchard, P., & Thacker, J. (2007). *Effective training: Systems, strategies, and practices* (3rd ed.). Upper Saddle River, NJ: Pearson Prentice Hall.

Blustein, D. (2006). *The psychology of working: A new perspective for career development, counseling, and public policy*. Mahwah, NJ: Erlbaum.

Boldry, J., & Gaertner, L. (2006). Separating status from power as an antecedent of intergroup perception. *Group Processes & Intergroup Relations, 9*, 377–400.

Borman, W. (2004). The concept of organizational citizenship. *Current Directions in Psychological Science, 13*, 238–241.

Boswell, W., Schipp, A., Payne, S., & Culbertson, S. (2009). Changes in newcomer job satisfaction over time: Examining the pattern of honeymoons and hangovers. *Journal of Applied Psychology, 94*, 844–858.

Bowman, J., & West, J. (2007). Lord Acton and employment doctrines: Absolute power and the spread of at-will employment. *Journal of Business Ethics, 74*, 119–130.

Brannon, L., Hershberger, P., & Brock, T. (1999). Timeless demonstrations of Parkinson's first law. *Psychonomic Bulletin & Review, 6*, 148–156.

Brehm, J. (1966). *A theory of psychological reactance*. New York: Academic Press.

Brewer, M. (2007). The importance of being "We": Human nature and intergroup relations. *American Psychologist, 62*, 728–738.

Brislin, R. (1981). *Cross-cultural encounters: Face-to-face interactions*. Elmsford, NY: Pergamon.

Brislin, R. (1991). *The art of getting things done: A practical guide to the use of power*. New York: Praeger.

Brislin, R. (2000). *Understanding culture's influence on behavior*, 2nd ed. Fort Worth, TX: Harcourt.

Brislin, R. (2001). *Power: Strategies and tactics*, Vol. 3, 1224–1228. In *The Corsini encyclopedia of psychology and behavioral science* (3rd ed.), eds. W. Craighead & C. Nemerof. New York: Wiley.

Brislin, R. (2008). *Working with cultural differences: Dealing effectively with diversity in the workplace*. Westport, CT: Greenwood.

Brislin, R., & Yoshida, T. (1994). *Intercultural communication training: An introduction*. Thousand Oaks, CA: SAGE.

Brislin, R., MacNab, B., Worthley, R., Kabigting, J., & Zukis, B. (2005). Evolving perceptions of Japanese workplace motivation: An employee-manager comparison. *International Journal of Cross-Cultural Management, 5*, 87–104.

Brown, K. G. (2005). Examining the structure and nomological network of trainee reactions: A closer look at "smile sheets." *Journal of Applied Psychology, 90*, 991–1001.

Buss, D. (2008). *Evolutionary psychology: The new science of the mind* (3rd ed.). Boston: Allyn & Bacon.

Bryce, T. (2006). Parkinson's law in IT. *Ezine articles*. Available at http://Ezine Articles.com/?expert=Tim_Bryce.

Butler, B., & Purchase, S. (2004). Personal networking in Russian post-Soviet life. *Research and Practice in Human Resource Management, 12*, 34–60.

Butters, J. (2005). Promoting healthy choices: The importance of differentiating between ordinary and high-risk cannabis use among high-school students. *Substance Use & Misuse, 46*, 845–855.

Carnall, C. (1990). *Managing change in organizations*. Englewood Cliffs, NJ: Prentice-Hall.

Carnegie, D. (1981). *How to win friends and influence people* (Rev. Ed.). NewYork: Pocket Books.

Chiaburu, D., & Marinova, S. (2005). What predicts skill transfer? An exploratory study of goal orientation, training self-efficacy and organizational supports. *International Journal of Training and Development, 9*, 110–123.

Choo, D. (2004, September). Local style for lolos. *Hawaii Business Magazine, 50*, 7–14.

Christie, R., & Geis, F. (1970). *Studies in Machiavellianism*. San Diego, CA: Academic Press.

Chu, P., Spires, E., Farn, C., & Sueyoshi, T. (2005). Decision processes and use of decision aids: Comparing two closely related nations in East Asia. *Journal of Cross-Cultural Psychology, 36*, 304–320.

Cialdini, R. B. (2001). *Influence: Science and practice* (4th ed.). Boston: Allyn & Bacon.

Cingoz-Ulu, B., & Lalonde, R. (2007). The role of culture and relational context in interpersonal conflict: Do Turks and Canadians use different conflict management strategies? *International Journal of Intercultural Relations, 31*, 443–458.

Cohen, S., & Janicki-Deverts, D. (2009). Can we improve our physical health by altering our social networks. *Perspectives on Psychological Science, 4*, 375–378.

Cohen, T., & Insko, C. (2008). War and peace: Possible approaches to reducing intergroup conflict. *Perspectives on Psychological Science, 3*, 87–93.

Coleman, V., & Borman, W. (2000). Investigating the underlying structure of the citizenship performance domain. *Human Resource Management Review, 10*, 25–44.

Connolly, T., & Zeelenberg, M. (2002). Regret in decision making. *Current Directions in Psychological Science, 11*, 212–216.

Cortes, A. (2000). Business protocol: A public relations approach. *Corporate Communications. 5*, 140–143.

Crick, B. (1982). *In defence of politics* (2nd ed.). Middlesex, UK and New York: Penguin.

Crosby, F. (2004). *Affirmative action is dead: Long live affirmative action*. New Haven, CT: Yale University Press.

Cummins, D. (2005). Dominance, status, and social hierarchies. In *The handbook of evolutionary psychology*, ed. D. Buss, 676–697. New York: Wiley.

Cummins, L., Nadorff, M., & Kelly, A. (2009). Winning and positive affect can lead to reckless gambling. *Psychology of Addictive Behaviors, 23*, 287–294.

Dahling, J., Whitaker, B., & Levy. P. (2009). The development and validation of a new Machiavellianism Scale. *Journal of Management, 35*, 219–257.

Dangerfield, R. (2004). *It's not easy being me*. New York: Harper-Collins.

Daniels, K., Hartley, R., & Travers, C. (2006). Beliefs about stressors alter stressors' impact: Evidence from two experience-sampling studies. *Human Relations, 59*, 1261–1285.

D'Aprix, R. (2009). *The credible company: Communicating with today's skeptical workforce.* San Francisco: Jossey-Bass.

DeBell, C. (2006). What all applied psychologists should know about work. *Professional Psychology: Research and Practice, 37,* 325–333.

De Cuyper, N., Notelaers, G., & De Witte, H. (2009). Job insecurity and employability in fixed-term contractors, agency workers, and permanent workers: Associations with job satisfaction and affective organizational commitment. *Journal of Occupational Health Psychology, 14,* 193–205.

De Dreu, C. (2005). A PACT against conflict escalation in negotiation and dispute resolution. *Current Directions in Psychological Science, 14,* 149–152.

Denhaerinck, P., Leyens, J., & Yzerbyt, V. (1989). The dilution effect and group membership: An instance of the pervasive impact of outgroup homogeneity. *European Journal of Social Psychology. 19,* 243–250.

Denhardt, R., Denhardt, J., & Aristigueta, M. (2009). *Managing human behavior in public and private organizations* (2nd ed.). Thousand Oaks, CA: SAGE.

Denrell, J. (2007). Adaptive learning and risk taking. *Psychological Review, 114,* 177–187.

Diener, D., & Diener, C. (1996). Most people are happy. *Psychological Science, 7,* 181–185.

Diener, E. (Ed). (2009). *Culture and well-being: The collected works of Ed Diener. Social indicators research series.* New York: Springer Science.

Diener, E., Lucas, R., & Scollon, C. (2006). Beyond the hedonic treadmill: Revisions to the adaptation theory of well-being. *American Psychologist, 61,* 305–314.

Diener, E., & Seligman, M. (2004). Beyond money: Toward an economy of well-being, *Psychological Science in the Public Interest, 5,* 1–31.

Dierdorff, E., Rubin, R., & Morgeson, F. (2009). The milieu of managerial work: An integrative framework linking work context to role requirements. *Journal of Applied Psychology, 94,* 972–988.

DiFonzo, N., & Bordia, P. (2007). *Rumor psychology: Social and organizational approaches.* Washington, DC: American Psychological Association.

Dixon, J., Durrheim, K., & Tredoux, C. (2005). Beyond the optimal contact strategy: A reality check for the contact hypothesis. *American Psychologist, 60,* 697–711.

Doest, L., Maes, S., Gebhardt, W., & Koelewijn, H. (2006). Personal goal facilitation through work: Implications for employee satisfaction and well being. *Applied Psychology: An International Review, 55,* 192–219.

Drory, A., & Romm, T. (1990). The definition of organizational politics: A review. *Human Relations, 43,* 1333–1354.

Duffy, S., & Crawford, L. E. (2008). Primacy or recency effects in forming inductive categories. *Memory & Cognition, 36,* 567–577.

Eisenberg, E. (2007). *Strategic ambiguities: Essays on communication, organization, and identity.* Thousand Oaks, CA: SAGE.

Ellis, A., Bell, B., Ployhart, R., Hollenbeck, J., & Ilgen, D. (2005). An evaluation of generic teamwork skills training with action teams: Effects on cognitive and skill-based outcomes. *Personnel Psychology, 58,* 641–72.

Ely, R., & Thomas, D. (2001). Cultural diversity at work: The effects of diversity perspectives on work group processes and outcomes. *Administrative Science Quarterly, 46,* 229–273.

Erev, I., Glozman, I., & Hertwig, R. (2008). What impacts the impact of rare events? *Journal of Risk Uncertainty, 36*, 153–177.

Erez, M., & Shokef, E. (2008). The culture of global organizations. In *The handbook of cross-cultural management research,* eds. P. Smith, M. Peterson, & D. Thomas, 285–300. Thousand Oaks, CA: SAGE.

Farh, L., Hackett, R., & Chen, Z-J. (2008). Organizational citizenship behavior in the global context. In *The handbook of cross-cultural management research,* eds. P. Smith, M. Peterson, & D. Thomas, 165–184. Thousand Oaks, CA: SAGE.

Fassinger, R. (2008). Workplace diversity and public policy: Challenges and opportunities for psychology. *American Psychologist, 63*, 252–268.

Feeney, J. (2006). Studying close relationships: Methodological challenges and advances. In *Close relationships: Functions, forms, and processes,* P. Noller & J. Feeney, 49–63. Hove, UK: Psychology Press/Taylor & Francis.

Felker, C. (Ed.). (1969). *The power game.* New York: Simon & Schuster.

Ferreira, M., Garcia-Marques, L., Sherman, S., & Sherman, J. (2006). Automatic and controlled components of judgment and decision making. *Journal of Personality and Social Psychology, 91*, 797–813.

Festinger, L. (1957). *A theory of cognitive dissonance.* Evanston, IL: Row, Petersen.

Fiedler, K. (2000). Beware of samples! A cognitive-ecological sampling approach to judgment biases. *Psychological Review, 107*, 659–676.

Fischer, R. (2008). Organizational justice and reward allocation. In *The handbook of cross-cultural management research,* eds. P. Smith, M. Peterson, & D. Thomas, 135–150. Thousand Oaks, CA: SAGE.

Fischer, R., & Ury, W. (1983). *Getting to yes: Negotiating agreement without giving in.* New York: Penguin Books.

Foa, U. (1971). Interpersonal and economic resources. *Science, 171*, 345–351.

Foa, U., & Chemers, M. (1967). The significance of role behavior differentiation for cross-cultural interaction training. *International Journal of Psychology, 2*, 45–57.

Foo, M. D., Uy, M., & Baron, R. (2009). How do feelings influence effort: An empirical study of entrepreneurs' affect and venture effort. *Journal of Applied Psychology, 94*, 1086–1094.

Forgas, J. (2008). Affect and cognition. *Perspectives on Psychological Science, 3*, 94–101.

Fredrickson, B. (1998). What good are positive emotions? *Review of General Psychology, 2*, 300–319.

Fredrickson, B., & Losada, M. (2005). Positive affect and the complex dynamics of human functioning. *American Psychologist, 60*, 678–686.

French, J., & Raven, B. (1959). The bases of social power. In *Studies of social power,* ed. D. Cartwright, 150–167. Ann Arbor, MI: Institute for Social Research.

Fukuyama, F. (1995). *Trust: The social virtues and the creation of prosperity.* New York: Free Press.

Furnham, A. (2002). Managers as change agents. *Journal of Change Management, 3*, 21–29.

Gagne, M., & Forest, J. (2008). The study of compensation systems through the lens of self-determination theory: Reconciling 35 years of debate. *Canadian Psychology, 49*, 225–232.

Gelenberg, A. (2009). E-etiquette. *Journal of Clinical Psychiatry, 70*, 103.

Gendolla, G., & Wicklund, R. (2009). Self-focused attention, perspective-taking, and false consensus. *Social Psychology, 40*, 66–72.

George, G. (2000). Emotions and leadership: The role of emotional intelligence. *Human Relations, 53*, 1027–1055.

Gibson, S. (2005). On judgment and judgmentalism: How counselling can make people better. *Journal of Medical Ethics, 31*, 575–577.

Gladwell, M. (2000). *The tipping point*. New York: Little, Brown.

Goldin-Meadow, S. (2006). Talking and thinking with our hands. *Current Directions in Psychological Science, 15*, 34–39.

Goldstein, D., & Gigerenzer, G. (2002). Models of ecological rationality: The recognition heuristic. *Psychological Review, 109*, 75–90.

Goldstone, R., Roberts, M., & Gureckis, T. (2008). Emergent processes in group behavior. *Current Directions in Psychological Science, 17*, 10–15.

Goleman, D. (1997). *Emotional intelligence*. New York: Bantam.

Grant, A., & Mayer, D. (2009). Good soldiers and good actors: Prosocial and impression management motives as interactive predictors of affiliative citizenship behaviors. *Journal of Applied Psychology, 94*, 900–912.

Greenberg, J. (1990). Organizational justice: Yesterday, today, and tomorrow. *Journal of Management, 16*, 399–432.

Greenberg, J. (1997). *The quest for justice on the job*. Thousand Oaks, CA: SAGE.

Greenberg, J., & Baron, R. (2008). *Behavior in organizations*, 9th ed. Upper Saddle River, NJ: Pearson.

Griffin, P., & Ouellett, M. (2007). Facilitating social justice education courses. In *Teaching for diversity and social justice*, 2nd edition, eds. M. Adams, L. Bell, & P. Griffin, 89–113. New York: Routledge.

Grout, J., & Fisher, L. (2007). *What do leaders really do? Getting under the skin of what makes a great leader tick*. Chichester, UK: Capstone/Wiley.

Gu, F., Hung, K., & Tse, D. (2008). When does Guanxi matter? Issues of capitalization and its dark sides. *Journal of Marketing, 72*, 12–28.

Gudykunst, W. (1983). Uncertainty reduction and the predictability of behavior in low- and high-context cultures: An exploratory study. *Communication Quarterly, 31*, 49–55.

Gupta, R., Derevensky, J., & Ellenbogen, S. (2006). Personality characteristics and risk-taking tendencies among adolescent gamblers. *Canadian Journal of Behavioural Science, 38*, 201–213.

Hackman, J., & Oldman, G. (1980). *Work redesign*. Reading, MA: Addison-Wesley.

Halbesleben, J., Wheeler, A., & Buckley, M. (2007). Understanding pluralistic ignorance in organizations: Application and theory. *Journal of Managerial Psychology, 22*, 65–83.

Halevy, N., & Sagiv, L. (2008). Teams within and across cultures. In *The Handbook of Cross-Cultural Management Research*, eds. P. Smith, M. Peterson, & D. Thomas, 253–268. Thousand Oaks, CA: SAGE.

Hall, E. (1959). *The silent language*. New York: Fawcett.

Hall, E. (1966). *The hidden dimension*. Garden City, NY: Doubleday.

Hammer, M. (1997). Negotiating across the cultural divide: Intercultural dynamics in crisis incidents. In *Dynamic processes of crisis negotiation*, eds. R. Rogan, M. Hammer, & C. Van Zandt, 9–24. Westport, CT: Praeger.

Haskard, K., Williams, S., DiMatteo, M. R., Heritage, J., & Rosenthal, R. (2008). The provider's voice: Patient satisfaction and the content-filtered speech of nurses and physicians in primary medical care. *Journal of Nonverbal Behavior, 32*, 1–20.

He, X., & Mittal, V. (2007). The effect of decision risk and project stage on escalation of commitment. *Organizational Behavior and Human Decision Processes, 103*(2), 225–237.

Henley, W. (1897). *The complete poetical works of Robert Burns.* Boston: Houghton Mifflin.

Hersey, P., & Blanchard, K. (1988). *Management of organizational behavior.* Englewood Cliffs, NJ: Prentice-Hall.

Herzberg, F., Mausner, B., & Snyderman, B. (1959). *The motivation to work.* New York: Wiley.

Hinde, R. (Ed.) (1972). *Non-verbal behavior.* Cambridge: Cambridge University Press.

Hodgkinson, G., & Healey, M. (2008). Cognition in organizations. *Annual Review of Psychology, 59*, 387–417.

Hofstede, G. (2001). *Culture's consequences: Comparing values, behaviors, institutions, and organizations across nations,* 2nd ed. Thousand Oaks, CA: SAGE.

Hogarth, R. M., & Karelaia, N. (2007). Heuristic and linear models of judgment: Matching rules and environments. *Psychological Review, 114*, 733–758.

Hollander, E. (1992). Leadership, followership, self, and others. *Leadership Quarterly, 3*, 43–54.

Holmes, T., & Rahe, R. (1967). The social readjustment rating scale. *Journal of Psychosomatic Research, 11*(2), 213–218.

Homans, G. (1950). *The social group.* New York: Harcourt.

Hong, L. (1978). Risky shift and cautious shift: Some direct evidence on the culture-value theory. *Social Psychology, 41*, 342–346.

House, R., Hanges, P., Javidan, M., Dorfman, P., & Gupta, V. (Eds.) (2004). *Culture, leadership, and organizations: The Globe study of 62 societies.* Thousand Oaks, CA: SAGE.

Houston, P., Blankstein, A., & Cole, R. (2010). *Leadership for family and community development.* Thousand Oaks, CA: Corwin Press.

Howard, A. (1964). *Ain't no big thing.* Honolulu: University of Hawaii Press.

Hsee, C., & Rottenstreich, Y. (2004). Music, pandas, and muggers: On the affective psychology of value. *Journal of Experimental Psychology: General, 133*, 23–30.

Huang, X. (2008). Motivation and job satisfaction across nations: How much do we really know? In *The handbook of cross-cultural management research,* eds. P. Smith, M. Peterson, & D. Thomas, 77–93. Thousand Oaks, CA: SAGE.

Hyun, J. (2005). *Breaking the bamboo ceiling: Career strategies for Asians.* New York: HarperCollins.

Illies, R., Fulmer, I., Spitzmuller, M., & Johnson, M. (2009). Personality and citizenship behavior: The mediating role of job satisfaction. *Journal of Applied Psychology, 94*, 945–959.

Iyengar, S. S., Wells, R. E., & Schwartz, B. (2006). Doing better but feeling worse—looking for the "best" job undermines satisfaction. *Psychological Science, 17*, 143–150.

Jandt, F. (1998). *Intercultural communication*, 2nd ed. Thousand Oaks, CA: SAGE.

Jang, S. (2009). The relationships of flexible work schedules, workplace support, supervisory support, work-life balance, and the well-being of working parents. *Journal of Social Service Research, 35*, 93–104.

Janis, I. (1982). *Victims of groupthink* (2nd ed.). Boston: Houghton Mifflin.

Johnson, D., & Hoopes, D. (2003). Managerial cognition, sunk costs and the evolution of industry structure. *Strategic Management Journal, 24*, 1057–1058.

Jones, R., & Brehm, J. (1970). Persuasiveness of one- and two-sided communications as a function of awareness that there are two sides. *Journal of Experimental Social Psychology, 6*, 47–56.

Judge, T., Ilies, R., & Colbert, A. (2004). Intelligence and leadership: A quantitative review and test of theoretical propositions. *Journal of Applied Psychology, 89*, 542–552.

Kahneman, D. (2003). A perspective on judgment and choice: Mapping bounded rationality. *American Psychologist, 58*, 696–720.

Kahneman, D., & Tversky, A. (2000). *Choices, values, and frames*. New York: Cambridge University Press.

Karnes, R. (2009). A change in business ethics: The impact on employer–employee relations. *Journal of Business Ethics, 87*, 189–197.

Kassam, K., Gilbert, D., Swencionis, J., & Wilson, T. (2009). Misconceptions of memory: The Scooter Libby effect. *Psychological Science, 20*, 551–552.

Kaushal, R., & Kwantes, C. (2006). The role of culture and personality in choice of conflict management strategy. *International Journal of Intercultural Relation, 30*, 579–603.

Kelley, H. (1967). Attribution theory in social psychology. In *Nebraska symposium on motivation*. Ed. D. Levine, 192–240. Lincoln: University of Nebraska Press.

Kelley, H. (1972). Attribution in social interaction. In *Attribution: Perceiving the causes of behavior*, eds. H. Kelley, R. Nisbett, S. Valins, & B. Weiner, 1–26. Morristown, NJ: General Learning Press.

Kelman, H. C. (1958). Compliance, identification, and internalization: Three processes of attitude change. *Journal of Conflict Resolution, 2*, 51–60.

Kelman, H. (2006). Interests, relationships, identities: Three central issues for individuals and groups in negotiating their social environment. *Annual Review of Psychology, 57*, 1–26.

Kesebir, P., & Diener, E. (2008). In pursuit of happiness: Empirical answers to philosophical questions. *Perspectives on Psychological Science, 3*, 117–125.

Khan, S., & Liu, J. (2008). Intergroup attributions and ethnocentrism in the Indian subcontinent: The ultimate attribution error revisited. *Journal of Cross-Cultural Psychology, 39*, 16–36.

Kim, H., Sherman, D., & Taylor, S. (2008). Culture and social support. *American Psychologist, 63*, 518–526.

Kinicki, A., & Williams, B. (2008). *Management: A practical approach* (3rd ed.). Boston: McGraw-Hill.

Kipnis, D. (1976). *The powerholders*. Oxford, UK: University of Chicago Press.

Kipnis, D. (2006). Does power corrupt? In *Small groups: Key readings in social psychology*, eds. J. Levine & R. Moreland, 177–186. New York: Psychology Press.

Kogan, N. (2002). Careers in the performing arts: A psychological perspective. *Creativity Research Journal, 14*, 1–16.

Kogan, N., & Wallach, M. (1964). *Risk taking: A study in cognition and personality*. New York: Holt.

Kurzman, P. (2009). Labor–social work collaboration: Current and historical perspectives. *Journal of Workplace Behavioral Health, 24*, 6–20.

Lambert, A., Chasteen, A., Payne, B. K., & Shaffer, L. (2004). Typicality and group variability as dual moderators of category-based inferences. *Journal of Experimental Social Psychology, 40*, 708–722.

Lambert, S. (2008). Passing the buck: Labor flexibility practices that transfer risk onto hourly workers. *Human Relations, 61*, 1203–1227.

Lammers, J., & Stapel, D. (2009). How power influences moral thinking. *Journal of Personality and Social Psychology, 97*, 279–289.

LaPierre, R. (1934). Attitude and action. *Social Forces, 13*, 230–237.

Lazarova, M., & Lowe, M. (2008). Work and family: Cross-national and international contexts. In *The handbook of crosscultural management*, eds. P. Smith, M. Peterson, & D. Thomas, 185–200. Thousand Oaks, CA: SAGE.

Lazarus, R. (1991). *Emotion and adaptation*. New York: Oxford University Press.

Lazarus, R., & Folkman, S. (1984). *Stress, adaptation, and coping*. New York: Springer.

Lewicki, R., Saunders, D., & Barry, B. (2006). *Negotiation* (5th ed.). New York: McGraw-Hill/Irwin.

Liddle, E., Scerif, G., Hollis, C., Batty, M., Groom, M., Liotti, M., & Liddle, P. (2009). Looking before you leap: A theory of motivated control of action. *Cognition, 112*, 141–158.

Lilienfeld, S., Ammirati, R., and Landfield, K. (2009). Giving debiasing away: Can psychological research on correcting social errors promote human welfare. *Perspectives on Psychological Science, 4*, 390–398.

Lim, J., & Guo, X. (2008). A study of group support systems and the intergroup setting. *Decision Support Systems, 45*, 452–460.

Lipscomb, R., Totten, J., Cook, R., & Lesch, R. (2007). Cellular phone etiquette among college students. *International Journal of Consumer Studies, 31*, 46–56.

Littrell, R. (2007). Influences on employee preferences for empowerment practices by "the ideal" manager in China. *International Journal of Intercultural Relations, 31*, 87–110.

Locke, E. A., & Latham, G. P. (1984). *Goal setting: A motivational technique that works!* Englewood Cliffs, NJ: Prentice-Hall.

Locke, E., & Latham, G. (1990). A theory of goal setting and task performance. Englewood Cliffs, NJ: Prentice Hall.

London, M. (2001). *Leadership development*. Mahwah, NJ: Erlbaum.

Machiavelli, N. (1940). *The Prince. The Discourses*. New York: Modern Library.

Marquardt, M., Leonard, H. S., Freedman, A., & Hill, C. (2009). Leadership and organizational change in the 21st century. In *Action learning for developing leaders and organizations: Principles, strategies, and cases*, eds. M. Marquardt, H. S. Leonard, A. Freedman, & C. Hill, 3–20. Washington, DC: American Psychological Association.

Martin, J. (1999). Communication and interpersonal effectiveness: Skills training for older adults. *Educational Gerontology, 25,* 269–284.

Maslow, A. (1943). A theory of human motivation. *Psychological Review, 50,* 370–396.

McClelland, D. (1976). Sources of stress in the drive for power. In *Psychopathology and human adaptation,* ed. G. Serban, 247–270. New York: Plenum Press.

McClelland, D. (1985). *Human motivation.* Glenview, IL: Scott, Foresman.

McGregor, D. (1960). *The human side of enterprise.* New York: McGraw-Hill.

McGuire, W. (1985). Attitudes and attitude change. In *Handbook of social psychology,* 3rd ed., Vol. 2, eds. G. Lindzey & E. Aronson, 233–346. New York: Random House.

Mehrabian, A. (1968). Communication without words. *Psychology Today,* September, 53–55.

Merton, R. (1957). *Social theory and social structure* (Rev. Ed.). New York: Free Press.

Meyer, J., Salovey, P., & Caruso, D. (2008). Emotional intelligence: New ability or eclectic traits? *American Psychologist, 63,* 503–517.

Milgram, S. (1970). The experience of living in cities. *Science, 167,* 1461–1468.

Miller, D., & Ross, M. (1975). Self-serving biases in attribution of causality: Fact or fiction. *Psychological Bulletin, 82,* 213–225.

Miller, W., & Rose, G. (2009). Toward a theory of motivated interviewing. *American Psychologist, 64,* 527–537.

Mindess, A. (1999). *Reading between the signs: Intercultural communication for sign language interpreters.* Yarmouth, ME: Intercultural Press.

Mischel, W. (2004). Toward an integrative science of the person. *Annual Review of Psychology, 55,* 1–22.

Molinsky, A., Krabbenhoft, M., Ambady, N., & Choi, Y. (2005). Cracking the nonverbal code: Intercultural competence and gesture recognition across cultures. *Journal of Cross-Cultural Psychology, 36,* 283–303.

Moon, S. (2003). Personal talent. *High Ability Studies, 24,* 5–21.

Moore, J. (2000). Why is this happening? A causal attribution approach to work exhaustion consequences. *Academy of Management Review, 25,* 335–349.

Morreall, J. (1991). Humor and work. *Humor—International Journal of Humor Research, 4,* 359–374.

Nakano, I. (2006). Silence and politeness in intercultural communication in university seminars. *Journal of Pragmatics, 38,* 1811–1835.

Natanovich, G., & Eden, D. (2008). Pygmalion effects among outreach supervisors and tutors: Extending sex generalizability. *Journal of Applied Psychology, 93,* 1382–1389.

Neustadt, D., Chamorro-Premuzic, T., & Furnham, A. (2006). The relationship between personality traits, self-esteem, and attachment at work. *Journal of Individual Differences, 27,* 208–217.

Noe, R., Hollenbeck, J., Gerhart, B., & Wright, P. (2008). *Human resource management: Gaining a competitive advantage* (6th ed.). New York: McGraw-Hill.

Oh, M., Chung, M-H., & Labianca, G. (2004). Group social capital and group-effectiveness: The role of informal socializing ties. *Academy of Management Journal, 47,* 893–906.

Okamura, J. (2008). *Ethnicity and inequality in Hawaii.* Philadelphia: Temple University Press.

Oldman, G., Hackman, J.R., & Pearce, J. (1976). Conditions under which employees respond positively to enriched work. *Journal of Applied Psychology, 61,* 395–403.

Olson, J., & Maio, G. (2003). Attitudes in social behavior. In *Handbook of psychology: Personality and social psychology,* Vol. 5, eds. T. Millon & M. Lerner, 299–325. New York: Wiley.

Osman-Gani, A., & Rockstuhl, T. (2009). Cross-cultural training, expatriate self-efficacy, and adjustments to overseas assignments: An empirical investigation of managers in Asia. *International Journal of Intercultural Relations. 33,* 277–290.

Oswald, M. & Grosjean, S. (2004). Confirmation bias. In *Cognitive illusions: A handbook on fallacies and biases in thinking, judgement and memory,* ed. R. Pohl, 79–96. East Sussex, UK: Psychology Press.

Pace, R. W. (2002). *Organizational dynamism: Unleashing power in the workforce.* Westport, CT: Quorum Books/Greenwood.

Park, H. S., Levine, T., Westerman, C., Foregger, S., & Orfgen, S. (2007). The effects of argument quality and involvement type on attitude formation and attitude change: A test of dual-process and social judgment predictions. *Human Communication Research, 33,* 81–102.

Parkinson, C. (1957). *Parkinson's law and other studies in administration.* Boston: Houghton Mifflin.

Pencavel, J. (2003). Review of worker participation: Lessons from the worker co-ops of the Pacific Northwest. *Personnel Psychology, 56,* 261–263.

Peter, L., & Hull, R. (1969). *The Peter principle.* New York: William Morrow.

Peterson, M., & Wood, R. (2008). Cognitive structures and processes in cross-cultural management. In *The handbook of cross-cultural management research,* eds. P. Smith, M. Peterson, & D. Thomas, 15–33. Thousand Oaks, CA: SAGE.

Pettigrew, T. (1998). Intergroup contact theory. *Annual Review of Psychology, 49,* 65–85.

Pettigrew, T. (2008). Future directions for intergroup contact theory and research. *International Journal of Intercultural Relations, 32,* 187–199.

Petty, R., & Brinol, P. (2008). Persuasion: From single to multiple metacognitive processes. *Perspectives on Psychological Science, 3,* 137–147.

Petty, R., Wheeler, C., Tormala, Z. (2003). Persuasion and attitude change. In *Handbook of psychology: Personality and social psychology,* Vol. 5. T. Millon & M. Lerner, 353–382. New York: Wiley.

Pinker, S. (2002). *The blank slate.* London: Penguin Classics.

Pistole, M. C., & Arricale, F. (2003). Understanding attachment: Beliefs about conflict. *Journal of Counseling and Development, 81,* 318–328.

Porter, L., & Lawler, E. (1968). *Managerial attitudes and performance.* Homewood, IL: Irwin.

Risen, J., Gilovich, T., & Dunning, D. (2007). One-shot illusory correlations and stereotype formation. *Personality and Social Psychology Bulletin, 33,* 1492–1502.

Robie, C., Brown, D. J., & Bly, P. (2008). Dysfunctional traits as moderators of the relations between the big five and promotability. *International Journal of Management, 25,* 131–139.

Robinson, J. (2001). The end of managed care. *Journal of the American Medical Association, 285*, 2622–2628.

Robinson, J., & Godbey, G. (1999). *Time for life: The surprising ways Americans use their time*. University Park: Penn State Press.

Rogers, E. (2003). *Diffusion of innovations*, 5th ed. New York: Free Press.

Rosenthal, R., & Jacobson, L. (1968). *Pygmalion in the classroom*. New York: Holt.

Rothton, C. (2008). Women, men and social class revisited: An assessment of the utility of a "combined" schema in the context of minority ethnic educational achievement in Britain. *Sociology, 42*, 691–708.

Rousseau, D. (2001). Schema, promise, and mutuality: The building blocks of the psychological contract. *Journal of Occupational and Organizational Psychology, 74*, 511–541.

Saavedra, R., & Kwun, S. (2000). Affective states in job characteristic theory. *Journal of Organizational Behavior, 21*, 131–146.

Sachau, D. (2007). Resurrecting the motivation-hygiene theory: Herzberg and the positive psychology movement. *Human Resource Development Review, 6*, 377–393.

Saviotti, P., & Pyka, A. (2004). Economic development by the creation of new sectors. *Journal of Evolutionary Economics, 14*, 1–35.

Schmidt, F., & Hunter, J. (2004). General mental ability in the world of work: Occupational attainment and job performance. *Journal of Personality and Social Psychology, 86*, 162–173.

Schnurr, S. (2009). Constructing leader identities through teasing at work. *Journal of Pragmatics, 41*, 1125–1138.

Sedikides, C., & Gregg, A. (2008). Self-enhancement: Food for thought. *Perspectives on Psychological Science, 3*, 102–116.

Seligman, M. (1975). *Helplessness: On depression, development, and death*. San Francisco: Freeman.

Seligman, M. (1991). *Learned optimism*. New York: Norton.

Shead, N., & Hodgins, D. (2009). Affect-regulation expectancies among gamblers. *Journal of Gambling Studies, 25*, 357–375.

Sherif, M. (1966). *In common predicament: Social psychology of intergroup conflict and cooperation*. New York: Houghton.

Sherif, M., Sherif, C., & Nebergall, R. (1965). *Attitudes and attitude change: The social judgment-involvement approach*. Philadelphia: Saunders.

Simon, H. (1978). Rationality as process and as product of thought. *The American Economic Review, 68*, 1–16.

Simons, T., Friedman, R., Liu, L., & McLean-Parks, J. (2007). Racial differences in sensitivity to behavioral integrity: Attitudinal consequences, in-group effects, and "trickle down" among Black and non-Black employees. *Journal of Applied Psychology, 92*, 650–665.

Simpson, J. (2007). Psychological foundations of trust. *Current Directions in Psychological Science, 16*, 264–268.

Singelis, T. (Ed.). (1998). *Teaching about culture, ethnicity, and diversity. Exercises and planned activities*. Thousand Oaks, CA: SAGE.

Smith, H. (1988). *The power game: How Washington works*. New York: Random House.

Smith, P. (2008). Indigenous aspects of management. In *The handbook of cross-cultural management research*, eds. P. Smith, M. Peterson, & D. Thomas, 319–332. Thousand Oaks, CA: SAGE.

Snibbe, A., & Markus, H. (2005). You can't always get what you want: Educational attainment, agency, and choice. *Journal of Personality and Social Psychology, 88*, 703–720.

Sternberg, R. (1986). *Intelligence applied*. New York: Harcourt.

Strauss, G. (2006). Worker participation: Some under-considered issues. *Industrial Relations: A Journal of Economy & Society, 45*, 778–803.

Tajfel, H. (1981). *Human groups and social categories*. Cambridge, UK: Cambridge University Press.

Tannen, D. (1990). *You just don't understand*. New York: Ballantine.

Tausig, M. (1982). Measuring life events. *Journal of Health and Social Behavior, 23*, 52–64.

Tetlock, P. (1985). Accountability: A social check on the fundamental attribution error. *Social Psychology Quarterly, 48*, 227–236.

Thibaut, J., & Kelley, H. (1959). *The social psychology of groups*. New York: Wiley.

Thomas, D., & Inkson, K. (2009). *Cultural intelligence* (2nd ed.). San Francisco: Berrett-Koehler.

Thomas, D., Ravlin, E., & Wallace, A. (1996). Effect of cultural diversity in work groups. *Research in Sociology of Organizations, 14*, 1–33.

Thompson, L. (1991). Information exchange in negotiation. *Journal of Experimental Social Psychology, 27*, 161–179.

Thompson, C., & Prottas, D. (2006). Relationships among organizational family support, job autonomy, perceived control, and employee well-being. *Journal of Occupational Health Psychology, 11*, 100–118.

Tooby, J., & Cosmides, L. (2005). Conceptual foundations of evolutionary psychology. In *The handbook of evolutionary psychology*, ed. D. Buss, 5–67. New York: Wiley.

Triandis, H. C. (1995). *Individualism and collectivism*. Boulder, CO: Westview Press.

Triandis, H. (2009). *Fooling ourselves: Self-deception in politics, religion, and terrorism*. Westport, CT: Greenwood.

Tversky, A., & Kahneman, D. (1973). Availability: A heuristic for judging frequency and probability. *Cognitive Psychology, 5*, 207–232.

Uchitelle, L. (2007). Employer-employee social contracts: Fashioning a new compact for workers. *Academy of Management Perspectives, 21(2)*, 5–9.

Van Hoye, G., & Lievens, F. (2009). Tapping the grapevine: A closer look at word-of-mouth as a recruitment source. *Journal of Applied Psychology, 94*, 341–352.

Van Iddekinge, C., Ferris, G., Perrewe, P., Perryman, A., Blass, F., & Heetderks, T. (2009). Effects of selection and training on unit-level performance over time: A latent growth modeling approach. *Journal of Applied Psychology, 94*, 829–843.

Van Vugt, M., Hogan, R., & Kaiser, R. (2008). Leadership, followership, and evolution: Some lessons from the past. *American Psychologist, 63*, 182–196.

Vassilopoulos, S. (2008). Social anxiety and ruminative self-focus. *Journal of Anxiety Disorders, 22*(5), 860–867.

Villere, M., & Hartman, S. (1990). The key to motivation is in the process: An examination of practical implications of expectancy theory. *Leadership & Organization Development Journal, 11*, i–iii.

Watson, W., & Michaelsen, M. (1984). Task performance information and leader participation behavior: Effect on leader–subordinate interaction, frustration, and future productivity. *Group & Organization Studies, 9*, 121–144.

Weakliem, D., & Frenkel, S. (2006). Morale and workplace performance. *Work and Occupations, 33*, 335–361.

Weber, E., & Johnson, E. (2009). Mindful judgment and decision making. *Annual Review of Psychology, 60*, 53–85.

Weick, K. (1984). Small wins: Redefining the scale of social problems. *American Psychologist, 39*, 40–49.

Wells, N., & Meche, M. (1999). Netiquette: A behavioral guide to electronic business communication. *Corporate Communications, 4*, 145–155.

Winter, D. (1973). *The power motive*. New York: Free Press.

Wright, S., & Taylor, D. (1999). Success under tokenism: Co-option of the newcomer and the prevention of collective protest. *British Journal of Social Psychology, 38*, 369–396.

Yukl, G. (2010). *Leadership in organizations*, 7th ed. Englewood Cliffs, NJ: Prentice Hall.

Zheng, W., Qu, Q., & Yang, B. (2009). Toward a theory of organizational cultural evolution. *Human Resource Development Review, 8*, 151–173.

Zimbardo, P. (1977). *Shyness: What it is, what to do about it*. New York: Perseus.

Zimbardo, P. (2007). *The Lucifer effect: Understanding how good people turn evil*. New York: Random House.

Zimbardo, P., & Leippe, M. (1991). *The psychology of attitude change and social influence*. New York: McGraw-Hill.

Zweigenhaft R., &. Domhoff, G. W. (1991). *Blacks in the white establishment? A study of race and class in America*. New Haven: Yale University Press.

Index

About the Author

Richard Brislin is a Shidler Distinguished Professor and Professor of Management and Department Chair, Shidler College of Business, University of Hawaii. Dr. Brislin is the co-developer of materials used in cross-cultural training programs (e.g., *Intercultural Interactions: A Practical Guide*, 2nd ed., 1996) and is author of a text in cross-cultural psychology (*Understanding Culture's Influence on Behavior*, 2nd ed., 2000). One of his books, *The Art of Getting Things Done: A Practical Guide to the Use of Power*, was a Book of the Month Club Selection in 1992. He is frequently asked to give workshops for American and Asian managers working on international assignments, and his training materials are widely used in various international organizations. One of his recent books is *Working with Cultural Differences: Dealing Effectively with Diversity in the Workplace* (2008).